PENGUIN BOOKS

THE FOUR-WEEK COUNTDOWN DIET

Namita Jain is a highly respected lifestyle and weight-management specialist and authority in the wellness industry. She holds prestigious international certifications in several fitness-related disciplines and has been actively involved in the wellness space for over twenty years, offering holistic guidance and teaching hundreds of students to get fitter, faster. She is a clinical fitness specialist at Bombay Hospital in Mumbai, structuring training programmes for patients with special needs, training the trainers and conducting specialized classes. Namita writes a variety of columns for leading newspapers and magazines in India, covering health issues such as nutrition, exercise and related topics.

She can be reached through her websites, www.liveactive.com and www.jaldifit.com

The Four-Week Countdown Diet

Now You Choose How You Lose

Namita Jain

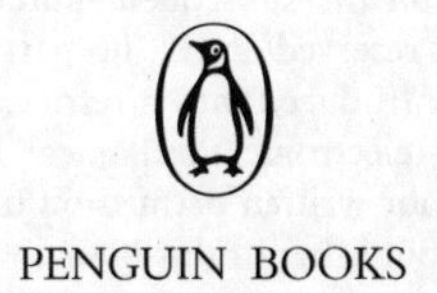

PENGUIN BOOKS

PENGUIN BOOKS
Published by the Penguin Group
Penguin Books India Pvt. Ltd, 11 Community Centre, Panchsheel Park, New Delhi 110 017, India
Penguin Group (USA) Inc., 375 Hudson Street, New York, New York 10014, USA
Penguin Group (Canada), 90 Eglinton Avenue East, Suite 700, Toronto, Ontario, M4P2Y3, Canada (a division of Pearson Penguin Canada Inc.)
Penguin Books Ltd, 80 Strand, London WC2R 0RL, England
Penguin Ireland, 25 St Stephen's Green, Dublin 2, Ireland (a division of Penguin Books Ltd)
Penguin Group (Australia), 250 Camberwell Road, Camberwell, Victoria 3124, Australia (a division of Pearson Australia Group Pty Ltd)
Penguin Group (NZ), 67 Apollo Drive, Rosedale, Auckland 0632, New Zealand
Penguin Group (South Africa) (Pty) Ltd, 24 Sturdee Avenue, Rosebank, Johannesburg 2196, South Africa

Penguin Books Ltd, Registered Offices: 80 Strand, London WC2R 0RL, England

First published by Penguin Books India 2011

10 9 8 7 6 5 4 3

ISBN 9780143067818

Typeset in Sabon by Eleven Arts, Delhi
Printed at Manipal Technologies Ltd., Manipal

Contents

Acknowledgements

This book has come to fruition thanks to the concerted efforts of my entire team. I am extremely grateful to my publisher, Penguin Books India, for giving me an opportunity to present my concept for a 'lifestyle' diet, THE FOUR-WEEK COUNTDOWN DIET. I have been encouraged and supported by their editorial team, led by Vaishali Mathur, all of whom have consistently offered valuable suggestions and insights at every stage of the book.

I am grateful to the film star Deepika Padukone for her quote, featured on the cover. She is the ultimate role model for a healthy, fit and active lifestyle.

I would like to acknowledge the inputs of my editor and creative consultant, Madhuri Iyer, for her contribution, including the titles and formats and the case studies.

I am indebted as well to Geeta Gopalakrishnan who has contributed in the capacity of creative consultant, offering her vast experience at the development and final stages of the book.

Last but certainly not least, I would like to thank my family and friends for their unstinting support.

PREFACE

'Ask me, I was overweight too . . .'

Plump. Obese. Chubby. Fat. Call it what you will, most of us know what it feels like to be on the heavy side. Speaking from experience, I understand how hard it is to shed those extra kilos. I have lived through the trials and tribulations of trying to lose weight. I have dealt with self-doubt, the highs, the lows, and sometimes, the hopelessness of it all.

But a voice inside urged me, encouraged me, to keep going. Not to give up. Today, I have managed to get to my ideal weight and stay there.

If I can do it, so can you.

As a wellness professional, I set an example by losing weight and keeping it off. This book now gives me the opportunity to share, quite literally, my ups and downs towards shedding the excess baggage!

To all you plus-size people out there, I have a message. I have put years of research into the weight-loss methods that you will find here. I have verified the efficacy of established diet plans and then, by trial and error, separated the facts from fiction. The result is a scientifically proven diet plan that really works.

In your fight against fat, don't for a moment imagine you are alone. I am with you all the way . . . we are a team. I am here to share my diet secrets and special tips. To show you simple diet solutions that you can work into your daily routine. And to help you win one of the most important battles of your life.

This is probably the easiest, most supportive diet plan you will ever attempt. I should add here, losing weight is not rocket science—just hang in there and believe in yourself. Yes, self-belief is your biggest weapon against weight loss. Use it!

Just like I got to my ideal weight with the help of my FOUR-WEEK COUNTDOWN DIET, you will too.

Good Luck!

SECTION I

THE FOUR-WEEK COUNTDOWN DIET

CHAPTER 1

AN INTRODUCTION TO DIETS

Why fads don't work

If you have picked up this book for yourself, congratulations. You have just taken your first step towards guaranteed weight loss.

Why do you want to lose weight? IDENTIFY YOUR X FACTOR

You undoubtedly have your own reasons for wanting to lose weight. It could be timely advice from your doctor, warning you to knock off the weight for health reasons. Maybe you plan to get married and want to look your best for the big day. Perhaps the 'middle-age spread' took its toll and you got overweight as the years rolled on. Or, the reason could quite simply be: you just can't bear to be fat any more.

Like you, and like every other overweight person on this planet, I had my demons to fight. As a plus-sized teenager, bursting out of my wardrobe was the least of my problems. Well-meaning aunts would look at me fondly and say, oh, puppy fat, it will disappear when you grow up. (These comments continued till I was twenty!) Friends in hip-hugging jeans sashayed their way through five years of college, while I trudged along the corridors knowing I needed to win the battle of the bulge.

Many of you will relate to what I was going through.

Apart from the personal trauma there could be social stigma attached to being fat. Airplane passengers could squirm when you make your way to the seat next to theirs. Elevator doors may shut faster when you approach. In a crowded bus . . . well, let's not go there!

Basically, you need to focus on one clear-cut 'reason why'. Find your very own motivator, the X factor that inspires you to lose weight. Let me emphasize here, if your mother is nagging you to shed the kilos, or if your husband wants a trophy wife, you will never be motivated enough to see the diet through. Because, when you are on a diet, no one else can motivate you. It's all about self-motivation.

It has to be you, and you alone, that makes the decision to go on a diet. First identify your reward, then work your way towards the goal. Once you zero in on your particular cause, hold on to it. Don't let go. Make it your life mission.

I had a client, a young man who was thoroughly fed up of being referred to as 'Mottu' all his life. Believe it or not, this was Arjun's sole incentive to shed twenty-odd kilos.

He did it.

So look deep inside, find your X factor.
And start getting the fat out of your system.

Once you are able to figure out what really drives your diet, what *your* motivating X factor is, you automatically have a reward in sight. This reward is the reason why you bother to make the effort in the first place.

Suddenly, your diet is not just drifting along, it has a destination. The reward is so attractive, so worthwhile, that you are prepared to go to any lengths for it.

***

Did you know choosing the right diet is as important as the diet itself?

This is probably not the first time that you are going on a diet. It may be your second or third attempt, or maybe you even lost count of the number of times you tried. You are not alone. You are among millions of dieters, across the world, who are in search of that magic formula that will miraculously transform their lives.

All of us begin our diets with a great deal of enthusiasm. However, as you and I know, most diets promise more than they deliver. This leads to disillusionment and, after a period of struggle, resignation. Your diet experience then turns into a vicious cycle of starving, overeating, feeling guilty and eating some more. You end up gaining all the weight you lost. What's worse, the more your weight shoots up, the more your self-esteem dives down.

If all this sounds painfully familiar, it's time do some serious introspection. It's time to take a call on the kind of diet plan you can live with. I mean really *live* with! To do that, you need a diet that fits in with your eating patterns and becomes a part of your regular routine. A diet that caters to *you*.

Working around the constraints of daily life, I have developed a unique diet plan that is easy to follow, without rigid rules or regulations, and yet it is a regimen that guarantees the most amazing results.

It's called the FOUR-WEEK COUNTDOWN DIET.

The FOUR-WEEK COUNTDOWN DIET is safe and simple and guarantees results within 4 weeks. With this plan, you don't just lose weight, you keep it off in the long run.

How did the FOUR-WEEK COUNTDOWN DIET come about? Being a health and wellness practitioner for over twenty years, I have come up-close and personal with hundreds of overweight people and their problems. I have seen my clients through thick and thin, no pun intended.

Moreover, having been overweight, I have dealt with many of these problems myself, not just in theory, but in practice. So, it was easier for me to rationalize the claims made by dieticians and exercise experts. Through my own experience, I was able to separate the facts from the fads. My journey towards weight loss has been one of discovery, experimentation and finally, a way forward, supported by the vast body of reference material I had collated through the years.

I have been looking for alternative, non-invasive methods to achieve weight loss. The process did not evolve overnight though. Initially, I made mistakes. It has taken me several years to fully understand how the body responds to diet and exercise. Over time, I found ways and means to rectify and reinvent certain techniques that needed to be modified. These tried-and-tested techniques are what I am now ready to share with you!

The good news is, you are not required to starve. On the contrary, you are expected to eat well and to get your daily supply of cereals, fruits and vegetables, and protein-rich foods within a balanced diet plan. This will make you shed weight *and* stay healthy, as you take full advantage of your wonderfully calibrated natural body responses.

I have always preferred a holistic, hands-on approach to good health, by integrating wellness into a healthy lifestyle. For dieters specifically, this means balanced nutrition and regular eating habits that ensure steady weight loss, as opposed to drastic calorie-cutting, or erratic eating patterns, which can lead to health problems in the long run.

The Atkins Diet advocates a high-protein intake. The GI Diet controls the body's glycemic index level. I am one hundred per cent behind my FOUR-WEEK COUNTDOWN DIET. This FOUR-WEEK COUNTDOWN DIET is based on a 1, 2, 3 formula.

The 1, 2, 3 Formula

What is the 1, 2, 3 Formula? 1 stands for cereal. 2 is the fruit and vegetable component. 3 comprises protein-rich foods. It is essential to include the 1, 2, 3 food groups in every meal, to ensure a balanced diet.

Why is a balanced diet so important? While there is no question that avoiding fats and sweets will help you lose weight, eliminating calories alone will not work. You need a balanced, nutritious diet plan, with a controlled calorie intake, as your safe, long-term solution to weight loss.

My FOUR-WEEK COUNTDOWN DIET comes with the calories pre-counted for you. So sit back and relax . . . thankfully, there's no need for complex mathematics in your head every time you put a morsel of food in your mouth!

'Working with the body' is a core value that I have extended across all my areas of expertise, in several wellness-related disciplines, ranging from clinical exercise to teenage diets.

Over the years, I have discovered that no two persons respond to a diet in quite the same manner. It can never be a one-size-fits-all solution. Every overweight person has his or her unique footprint, which must allow for a unique solution.

The FOUR-WEEK COUNTDOWN DIET is therefore all about choices. Food options are flexible, timings are adjustable. In fact, my FOUR-WEEK COUNTDOWN DIET is made to order . . . for you!

CHAPTER 2

Introducing!

THE FOUR-WEEK COUNTDOWN DIET

A week-by-week diet plan that allows you to be yourself

Welcome to the FOUR-WEEK COUNTDOWN. You are about to start a diet that does not feel like a diet. Let me introduce you to a friendly, flexible diet plan that allows you to be yourself. Over a four-week period, you will gradually slip into your diet, by incorporating one additional diet meal every week. At the end of week 4, the entire FOUR-WEEK COUNTDOWN DIET will become a part of your daily routine.

The idea is simple.

I'm sure you are with me when I say, starting a new diet is never a problem, but actually sticking to it is the challenge. Well, research supports your sentiments! It has been consistently proved that, by the second or third week, a dieter's will power weakens. The temptation to binge takes over. You give in to your cravings and, before you know it, your diet spins out of control.

Staying hungry is forbidden!

Time and again, I have seen dieters struggle with starvation and then succumb to all-they-can-eat binges. This syndrome is highly counter-productive. I have therefore structured a diet plan that does not permit you to be hungry. In fact, staying hungry is forbidden! Throughout the FOUR-WEEK COUNTDOWN, it is important to consume the prescribed portions at every meal and to maintain your eating pattern over the entire diet period.

And yes, you might be surprised to know that you are still going to lose weight. So how does it work? How do you eat six times a day, ensure your daily supply of nutrients, never go hungry, and yet get guaranteed weight loss results?

My 1, 2, 3 Formula gives you complete, balanced nutrition, by including one portion of cereal, one portion fruits and vegetables, and one protein-rich food option, in just the right quantities.

By adapting to your lifestyle, the FOUR-WEEK COUNTDOWN fits into your daily routine with well-planned meals and mini-meals all through the day. This means, even as you are on the COUNTDOWN, you can lead a fairly 'normal' life—you won't feel like an alien during the office lunch hour, or have to refuse dinner invitations because you're not allowed to eat!

The template I am presenting here is a break-up of your entire FOUR-WEEK COUNTDOWN DIET plan, using the 1, 2, 3 Formula. All your COUNTDOWN dinners, breakfasts, in-betweens and lunches are divided into the three balanced food groups—cereals, fruits and vegetables, and protein-rich foods—to ensure you lose weight without losing out on your health.

1. CEREAL: the body's main energy provider

2. FRUITS & VEGETABLES: rich in vitamins and minerals, high in fibre, help immunity and aid digestion
3. PROTEIN-RICH FOODS: the body's building blocks, working for repair and regeneration

INTERESTING FACT

India's cuisine is as rich and varied as the diverse Indian culture. But despite this diversity, there is a common uniting factor—the great Indian thali! The thali exemplifies all that is good in a balanced, well-rounded meal plan, offering complete nutrition. In much the same way, the 1, 2, 3 Formula too prescribes all-round nutrition for every meal.

The 1, 2, 3 Formula, that is a balanced food intake, gets your body's digestive enzymes to work on all the three food groups. This not only keeps the body satiated, it also provides the vital nutrients needed to keep it working at peak performance levels. (Conversely, eating large amounts of only one or two food groups can make you fidgety, irritable, inattentive and very often, sleepy and lethargic.)

Equally important, you learn to space out your food consumption at regular intervals. The logic here is, if you eat more often, you will speed up your metabolism, burn more calories and therefore, lose more weight. This is precisely why I encourage small, frequent meals, every three hours or so.

Apart from the logical explanation, there is a physiological reason why the 1, 2, 3 Formula works best for weight loss.

All foods burn calories during the digestive process. This process of burning calories is known as the thermic effect of food. But the interesting thing is, not all foods burn at the same rate! So if different foods have different 'burn rates', how can you make the most of this during your diet? My Formula shows you how.

1. Cereals produce a thermic effect, or burn rate, of 20 per cent, which is fairly high.

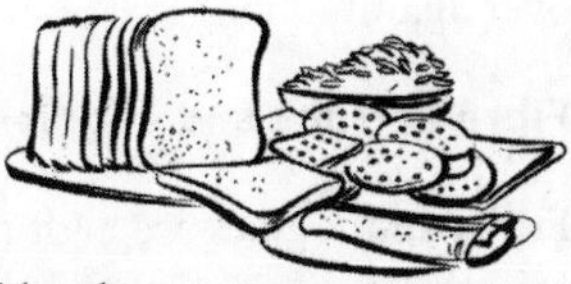

Cereals contain carbohydrates and are the body's main energy source. You need regular and controlled cereal portions to minimize swings in blood sugar levels and insulin levels. Your red blood cells and brain cells also depend on carbohydrates for energy.

However, a meal consisting primarily of cereals is not a balanced option. The excess unused energy from cereals makes you sluggish and ultimately, gets converted to fat.

On the other hand, giving up, or severely restricting cereals does not work either, because you are deprived of your energy requirements. Your body then has to derive its energy from the breakdown of muscle protein or muscle tissue. This deliberately induced state, known as gluconeogenesis, leads to muscle breakdown and deterioration in muscle strength.

2. Fruits and vegetables produce a thermic effect, or burn rate, of 20 per cent.

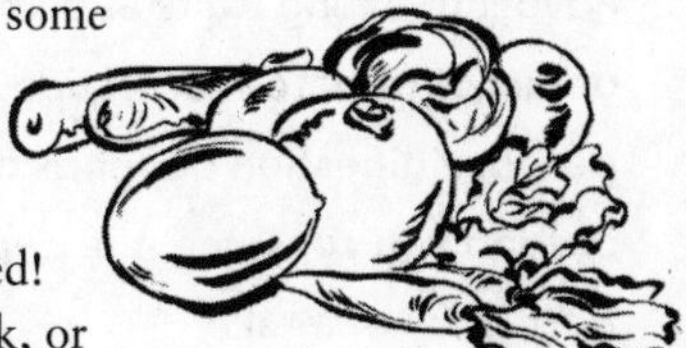

Now here's something interesting. Fruits and vegetables elicit the same thermic effect as cereals. But unlike cereals, fruits and veggies contain high levels of moisture, in some cases, a water content of up to 90 per cent. So, fruits and vegetables contain fewer calories, but require just as many calories to get digested! Some veggies, such as a celery stick, or a piece of cucumber, require as many calories to chew and digest as the total amount of calories they contain! This is like eating zero calories, obviously giving you a tremendous fat-burning advantage.

While fruits and veggies are a great source of vitamins and minerals, with great fat-burning properties, it is not practical to make a meal of this food group alone. A meal consisting only of these will get digested really fast and you will be starving all over again!

Fibre in fruits and veggies—how much is too much?

Fruits and veggies are high-fibre foods that work as cleansers, effectively eliminating the waste from the digestive system. As fibre passes through the digestive tract, it acts like a sponge, cleansing the waste matter and preventing constipation. Fibre softens the stools, making the rate of colonic transit easier.

Nutritionally speaking, it is good to eat about 35 gm of fibre every day. Start gradually, by adding a little more fibre to your diet. Loading up on fibre too quickly can cause abdominal discomfort. You can overdo fibre if you consume more than 50–60 gm per day. This may cause a decrease in absorption of certain vitamins and minerals such as zinc, iron and magnesium.

MYTH BUSTER

I am aware that many dieticians and nutritionists advocate eating fruits as a stand-alone item, because of 'uncomplicated' digestion. This makes little sense, because digestion depends on several factors: the type of food you consume, the quantity of food, and the frequency of intake.

In fact, all foods undergo a similar breakdown process in the digestive tract. So, rather than eat fruit alone, you are better off consuming fruit along with cereals and protein-rich foods, because the balanced intake keeps you fully satiated, and for a longer period of time.

You are therefore more easily able to maintain a two-and-a-half- to three-hour gap between meals without feeling famished, clearly explaining why there is no connection between eating fruits alone and weight loss.

3. Proteins elicit the highest thermic effect, up to 30 per cent.

This means that the energy, or calorie burn, during the digestion of protein is the highest. Protein also takes *more time* to digest and, as we well know, feeling full longer is a critical component for achieving lasting weight loss.

But like they say, you can't have too much of a good thing! The downside of consuming protein-rich foods in excess is that it is hard to digest and can strain the liver and kidneys.

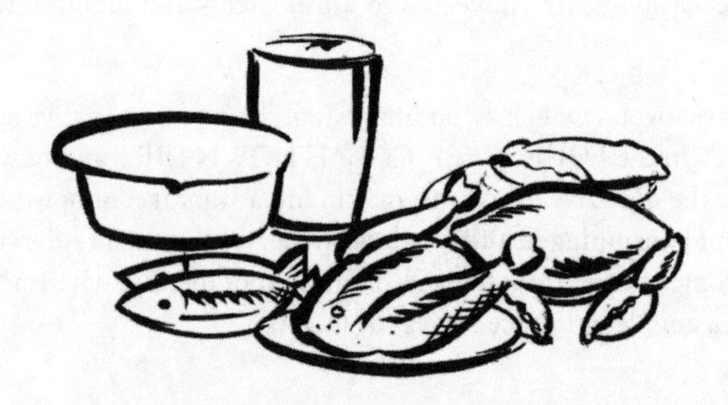

FAT FACT

Last but not the least, we come to fats. The thermic effect of fat is the lowest, a mere 3 per cent. Fats use the least number of calories when digested, which is one reason why eating fats results in easy weight gain. However, consuming a small quantity of fat is necessary, even when you are on a diet, as fat is essential for the absorption of fat-soluble vitamins and for the manufacture of essential hormones. Fat also helps you maintain healthy skin and hair.

Q: So how does digestion actually work?

A: The food goes into the stomach and the intestine and is broken down by enzymes in the body. It undergoes a process of digestion, absorption and elimination. The body absorbs its nutrients from multiple sources and, after eliminating waste products, stores the excess as fat. Cereals, fruit and vegetables are converted into glucose. Proteins are converted to amino acids and fats to fatty acids.

This basic overview helps you understand how your digestive system responds to the FOUR-WEEK COUNTDOWN DIET and how you can use the digestive process to maximum advantage. Simply put, it's all about consuming healthy, balanced meals at frequent intervals. A welcome change from the age-old notion of dieting, where a 'diet' means a couple of lettuce leaves for lunch.

The Thermic Effect of Food
is the metabolic rate at which food is digested

CEREALS	thermic effect	20%
FRUITS & VEGGIES	thermic effect	20%
PROTEIN-RICH FOODS	thermic effect	30%
FATS	thermic effect	3%

Bear in mind, however, while your FOUR-WEEK COUNTDOWN is friendly and flexible, it is still a diet. Quantities have to be limited. Certain high-fat foods have to be eliminated. So please do not build unrealistic expectations, but learn to work in tandem with your body, to make the most of the effort you will be putting in.

Let's put the facts on the table.

You will not lose weight overnight. It takes effort to lose weight. Exercise is an integral part of the weight loss programme too. You have to maintain a healthy lifestyle to keep the kilos off in the long term. In short, there is no free lunch!

During the FOUR-WEEK COUNTDOWN you will learn to adapt to a new style of eating and create new lifestyle habits. It is best to combine exercise and diet to effectively lose weight and stay fit. If, for some reason, you choose to follow the FOUR-WEEK COUNTDOWN without an exercise routine, you will definitely lose weight, but at a slower pace.

After the initial phase of the FOUR-WEEK COUNTDOWN, I have a Way Forward section. In that section I will share tips on how to stay on a maintenance plan and work towards further weight loss goals.

Before we get started on the FOUR-WEEK COUNTDOWN, I would like to quickly run through some typical questions my clients ask. I am sure the same queries are on your mind too. This little exercise will help you separate the facts from the fads, and the answers here might surprise you!

One of my clients, Benaifer Billimoria, was convinced that the more calories she cut, the more weight she would lose. She therefore tried to eliminate all fat from her diet.

That kind of thinking can actually hurt you. Cut your calories too far below 1200 a day and you'll end up slowing your metabolism, losing muscle mass and falling sick due to lack of immunity. The truth is, a very low-calorie, no-fat diet is as harmful as a high-fat diet.

Fat consumption should be greatly reduced, but never eliminated. Why are fats essential? They provide the body with energy and are needed to maintain healthy skin and hair. They are also responsible for transporting crucial fat-soluble vitamins A, D, E and K. In addition, some amounts of essential fatty acids are required for the manufacture of certain hormones.

Many clients want to know how much weight they can lose. Some think losing 2 kg a week is an easy target.

I tell such clients to get real! First of all, weight loss varies from person to person. On an average, you could lose anything between 2–4 kg in 4 weeks. In fact, it is advisable not to lose more than 4 kg a month. If you are on a crash diet, you may initially lose more weight, but that loss is mostly of lean muscle mass and water. It is therefore important to eat a balanced diet that gives you steady weight loss in terms of higher fat percentages, and not loss of water or muscle mass.

Factors such as genetic disposition, constitution, physical activity and food habits determine weight loss results. If you are already close to your ideal weight you will lose less, because the body has already reached its destination weight. A general thumb rule is, the more weight you need to lose, the faster you will shed it off!

So is it really possible to lose 1 kg a week?

Yes, it is. In general, your weight loss is directly related to your current Body Mass Index (BMI) and dietary habits. For example, on the COUNTDOWN diet, you create a calorie deficit of 300 to 700 calories per day. Exercise burns up another 250–300 calories, giving you a total deficit of 500 to 1000 calories in a day.

3500 calories burnt = 1 pound weight loss
7000 calories burnt = 2 pounds weight loss
(7 days @ 1000 calories burned per day)

Therefore in 7 days, or one week, you lose 2 lb which is approximately equal to 1 kg. Retaining this weight loss rate through the FOUR-WEEK COUNTDOWN adds up to a total weight loss of about 4 kg in one month.

Pilates is a fitness programme I teach, and one of my Pilates students, Kedar, was of the opinion that skipping meals would help him lose weight faster.

I had a hard time convincing him otherwise! I had to get Kedar to understand that skipping meals did not mean quicker weight loss. I told him about people who skipped breakfast and put on more weight. I gave him the scientific explanation for this. Hunger causes a drop in blood sugar levels and this, in turn, leads to food cravings. So you end up binge eating, grabbing all the calorie-packed foods you can lay your hands on.

Plus, when your body recognizes that food is scarce, it immediately starts preparing for 'famine' by stubbornly storing all the fat reserves you have!

On the other hand, if you make the effort to eat healthy, at regular intervals of two to three hours, your body knows there is a steady supply of food coming and finds no reason to store the excess fat.

Prachi Gupta, one of my group fitness class students, had tried several diets, but could not stick with anything. She complained about having to re-schedule her entire life to accommodate her diets.

I taught Prachi how to read her body clock and work with her body to accomplish her goals. She could eat every three hours, she could pick her food preferences, as long as she maintained the diet guidelines. Prachi learnt to eat a healthy, balanced diet, with all the essential nutrients included.

The main objective was to move away from a structured diet plan to a more flexible eating pattern that could be integrated into her lifestyle. Soon, Prachi started calling her regimen 'The Prachi Gupta Diet', because she was so completely in sync with it!

I get this question all the time: 'How often should I weigh myself? And what is the best time to weigh in?'

When on a diet, it is best to weigh yourself once a week. It is a good idea to weigh yourself first thing in the morning. Wear light clothing to ensure an accurate reading.

Another common diet-related question is the problem of constipation. Many of my new clients come in with this particular complaint.

In most cases, constipation is the result of a faulty diet. When you eat an excess of refined food, or do not get enough water, you are likely to suffer from constipation.

The body needs about 25 to 30 gm of fibre a day, to keep the digestive system functioning efficiently. This has to be consumed in the form of fresh fruits and vegetables, whole grains, pulses, sprouts and seeds. I encourage all my clients to consume non-refined foods and to ensure that their bodies get ample fluids through the day.

Remember, the combination of fibre and fluids is vital, because a high-fibre intake without sufficient fluids can result in constipation.

You may use a laxative like Esapgol if required. But first try to have a high-fibre diet to prevent constipation. Keep in mind that a sedentary lifestyle also slows down the bowels, so regular exercise goes a long way in reducing constipation.

I have lost count of the number of clients who come to me and insist on starting a 'high-protein diet'.

'High-protein' diets can lead to unpleasant side effects. Excess protein, just like excess carbohydrates, gets stored as fat. It also places undue stress on the liver and kidneys.

Moreover, on a daily basis, our bodies do not require more than 0.8–1 gm of protein per kilogram of body weight. Instead of fad diets, the only thing that really works, long term, is a balanced diet that caters to your body's nutritional requirements.

I have a friend, Rachel, a non-vegetarian, who just loves eating out. When she went on a diet, her first question was, 'Can I still eat out?'

Rachel looked so anxious, I was happy to reassure her! Eating out did not mean the end of her diet. She just had to learn to make better food choices. For example, she could request for foods to be steamed, baked or grilled instead of fried.

To keep dieters like Rachel on course, several substitute options could be ordered.

- baked or roasted fish and chicken, as opposed to buttered or fried alternatives
- salads could come with lemon dressing instead of mayonnaise
- mint chutney or salsa could work as the perfect substitute for creamy sauces
- tandoori food instead of rich gravy dishes
- roti instead of buttery naan

Sometimes, a married couple decides to go on a diet together. Naturally, this is a convenient option and also a great morale booster. But can it really work?

Yes it can. However, it's worth keeping in mind that men need an additional calorie allowance. This is because men have more testosterone, a hormone that promotes the development of muscle. More muscle means a higher metabolic rate and a greater ability to burn calories during exercise and at rest.

Men need to supplement this extra energy requirement by consuming an additional 150 calories per day. (The FOUR-WEEK COUNTDOWN factors this additional allowance for men in week 4 of the diet.)

As you begin your FOUR-WEEK COUNTDOWN, it makes sense to prepare, physically and mentally, for the weeks ahead.

The FOUR-WEEK COUNTDOWN cuts out erratic, extreme eating habits and helps you towards a safe, steady weight-loss plan. While most diets could deplete your body of energy or nutrients, the FOUR-WEEK COUNTDOWN gradually eases you into a whole new routine that nourishes your body as it melts away the extra kilos.

A vital first step is to understand your current eating pattern. Only when you become aware of your daily food habits, realize where you are going wrong and register your weaknesses, can you rectify the mistakes. Right? Once you figure this out, you know, with just a little tweaking, it's possible to completely revamp your eating habits and move towards healthier food choices.

So are you ready? Let the COUNTDOWN begin!

Through 4 weeks, the COUNTDOWN modifies one meal per week. In the first week, you start by trimming dinner. In the second week, while you continue with your COUNTDOWN dinners, you also modify your breakfast. In the third week, the in-between snacks, along with the diet dinner and breakfast, become part of your COUNTDOWN. By week four, lunch is also included, thereby incorporating your entire food consumption for the day.

Countdown Calendar

WEEK 1	Modify Dinner
WEEK 2	Modify Breakfast
WEEK 3	Modify In-Between Snacks
WEEK 4	Modify Lunch

The FOUR-WEEK COUNTDOWN works in sync with your body clock

The FOUR-WEEK COUNTDOWN uses your natural body clock to maximum advantage. The morning hours are when you are at your most active, with peaking energy levels. Towards the evening, you tend to slow down, so your body does not require as much energy as it did earlier in the day. It is therefore smart to distribute your calories wisely, by consuming more calories during the day than at night.

Why dinner has to be your first diet meal. If, like most people, dinner is your biggest meal of the day, you have a problem. Based on your metabolic activity, it should actually be your lightest meal.

Dinner time is a danger zone for your diet. Think about it. First comes the temptation of tucking into a nice, rich dinner. Soon after comes the equally enticing prospect of tucking yourself into bed. Please do not do it. I earnestly advise you to stay within your COUNTDOWN dinner guidelines and, at any cost, avoid sleeping on a full stomach. Thank you.

Make sure you clock in for breakfast. Breakfast has its own set of rules. Rules number one, two and three: breakfast should never be skipped. This is because, post-dinner, it has been a long gap until breakfast. Your body needs urgent replenishment now. So work with your body, giving it what it needs, and when it needs it.

The calories consumed during the morning hours are burned more easily and work their way out of your system. So make the most of breakfast!

Don't forget to snack round the clock. In-Between snacking is compulsory and yes, I will actually force you to snack all day! Your COUNTDOWN In-Betweens are a great way to lose weight, because, in order to digest the food, your metabolism automatically gets fired up into an energy burning mode.

Pick your In-Betweens based on the COUNTDOWN choices, so that you keep your energy levels cranked up from mid-morning all the way up to dinner time.

Bag, box or buffet, lunch is an important meal. Midday is when your body is going full throttle as you run through your daily routine. You can afford to eat a fairly substantial amount, to sustain your energy levels at this time of the day.

Even if you are on the go, try to sit down and enjoy your COUNTDOWN lunch. You will find varied menus on offer, to make lunch something to look forward to.

FOUR-WEEK COUNTDOWN

IN 10 SIMPLE STEPS

1 FIGURE OUT HOW MUCH
weight you need to lose—refer to
BMI Annexure

2 SLOT YOURSELF
into diet Plan Minimum, Plan Medium or
Plan Maximum based on weight loss goals

3 UNDERSTAND YOUR CURRENT
EATING PATTERN
for One-day Recall

4 PREPARE YOURSELF MENTALLY
for the 4 weeks ahead

5 MODIFY
dinner

6 MODIFY
breakfast

7 MODIFY
in-betweens

8 MODIFY
lunch

9 REFER TO WAY FORWARD
to figure out how to maintain your weight or lose more

10 TAKE UP REGULAR EXERCISE & NEW EATING HABITS
as a way of life

CHAPTER 3

DIET PLANS MINIMUM, MEDIUM AND MAXIMUM

Figure out how much weight you need to lose, then slot yourself based on your weight-loss goals

Now comes the most interesting part of your FOUR-WEEK COUNTDOWN. Unlike most diets, where one size fits all, the COUNTDOWN is designed keeping in mind that each of you has a different size and shape. The more you weigh, the more calories you need to burn. As you lose weight, the calories your body requires will also get reduced.

It's a little like shoe size. Just as you need a particular size of shoe, appropriate for your foot size, similarly, you need a 'diet size', depending on your weight and height. We don't all come in the same shape or size, so why must the entire diet universe be restricted to a single diet plan?

The more I thought about this, I knew I had to customize the COUNTDOWN to make it more relevant for a cross section of dieters. (Easier said than done!) I worked extensively, and used statistical figures, to arrive at my final three diet plans.

Plan Minimum	@ 1250 calories per day
Plan Medium	@ 1400 calories per day
Plan Maximum	@ 1550 calories per day

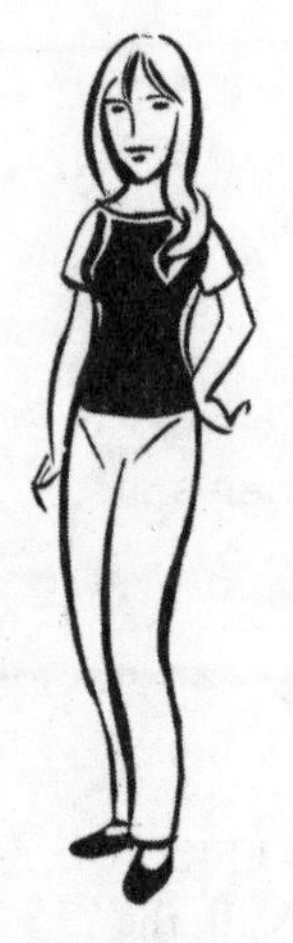

Plan Minimum

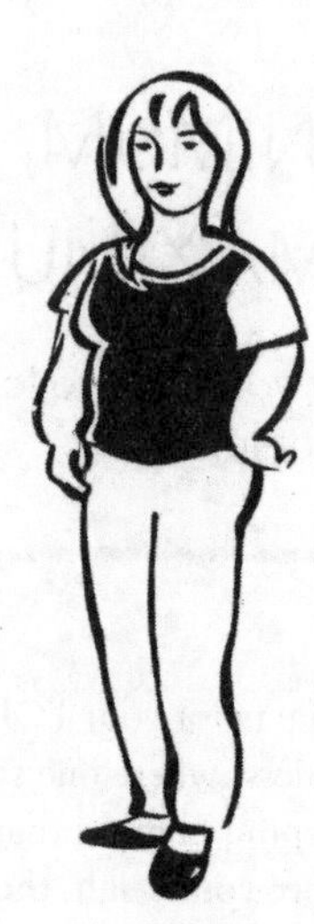

Plan Medium

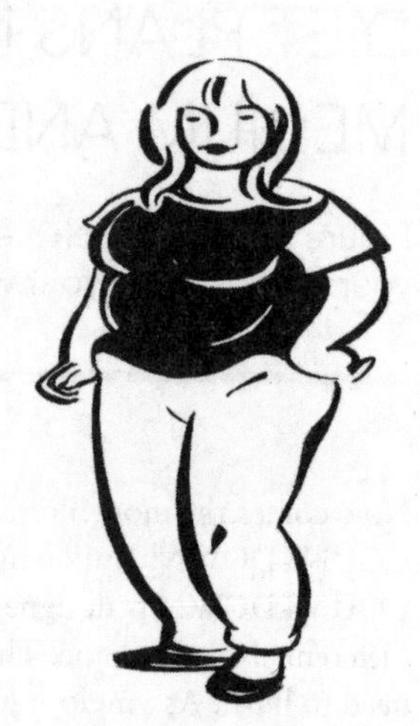

Plan Maximum

Because of genetic differences, men require a higher calorie intake, and *do not qualify* for the **Plan Minimum**. They have to slot themselves into **Plan Medium** or **Plan Maximum**.

Women can slot themselves into **Plan Minimum, Plan Medium** or **Plan Maximum**.

Aiming for a realistic target weight is a key factor in determining how much weight you need to lose. I call this the **Perfect-Fit Weight** because this is the weight at which your body feels most comfortable. Once you are aware of the number of kilos you need to shed, you can automatically slot yourself into the right Diet Plan—Minimum, Medium or Maximum.

MEN

Plan Medium

for men who need to lose up to 4 kg

Plan Maximum

for men who need to lose more than 5 kg

WOMEN

Plan Minimum

for women who need to lose up to 4 kg

Plan Medium

for women who need to lose between 5 and10 kg

Plan Maximum

for women who need to lose more than 11 kg

So what do you do if you do not know how much weight you need to lose?

And how do you determine your target weight or perfect-fit weight?

I have suggested a method here. This is covered in Annexure A: BODY MASS INDEX (BMI). The calculation is based on your BMI (your weight and height ratio). In addition, this section gives a detailed explanation of what the readings indicate.

However, if you have already managed to slot yourself in one of the three plans, you may omit Annexure A altogether. Once you slot yourself, please take time to follow the diet requirements of your selected plan. Annexure B has detailed charts and tables to help you understand the serving sizes of different food groups.

Keep in mind: *Familiarizing yourself with your selected diet plan is crucial to the successful completion of your COUNTDOWN.*

FOUR-WEEK COUNTDOWN PLUS POINTS

- Boosts metabolism and energy levels
- Helps you lose weight safely
- Revolves around your lifestyle and eating habits
- Encourages you to vary your food and menus
- Gives you a way forward at the end of 4 weeks for weight maintenance or further weight loss
- Shapes and tones your body

CHAPTER 4

ONE-DAY RECALL

How to understand your current eating pattern

This chapter is dedicated to preparing you for your COUNTDOWN.

You must keep in mind that there is no point following the FOUR-WEEK COUNTDOWN diet plan to perfection, and also indulging in all kinds of calorie-dense items through the day. To see results, it is vital to start controlling your intake from day one of your diet.

In your first week, although you are only following the COUNTDOWN for dinner, it is important to keep track of your other meals, so that you don't go overboard on your calories during the rest of the day. But how do you do this?

Start by taking a typical day in your life. (I specify a week day because, over the weekend, you are more likely to indulge and your record won't be consistent.) So say you choose a day mid-week, for example, a Wednesday. Keep a piece of paper handy and track your food consumption through the day. Jot down every last bit of food you consume, how much you eat, and when.

This record becomes your One-Day Recall.

From day one of your COUNTDOWN, your One-day Recall will help you to understand your eating patterns and cut down on indulgences. Use the following guidelines, an essential part of the COUNTDOWN, to keep you on track.

1. Attempt to eliminate all deep-fried foods; substitute fried foods with baked or roasted alternatives. For example, have your chicken roasted, or your fish grilled, instead of fried. Namkeens such as sev, papdi, khakra or chivda can all be had baked instead of fried.
2. Restrict sweets such as desserts, mithais, cakes and puddings. Whatever be your sweet consumption, REDUCE IT BY HALF. Try to choose healthier options like raisins, dates, dried figs or apricots, til ladoo or kurmura (puffed rice) chikki.
3. Go for coconut water or herbal tea instead of soft drinks.
4. Try to cut back on high-calorie fats such as cream, butter and oil. Get your palate to slowly adapt to dishes with a minimal amount of fat. If, for instance, you are having pasta, use a tomato-based sauce instead of a cream-based one.

By week 4 of the COUNTDOWN, you will have to reduce your fat intake to a maximum of two teaspoons a day. So try to gradually move towards that goal. You will discover, soon enough, that your roasted khakra with mint chutney is a viable option to the greasy pakora you had in mind!

Let me remind you, once again, that the guidelines mentioned here should not make you a slave to your diet. The COUNTDOWN is structured to accommodate you, your needs, your lifestyle. Apart from certain food items that are detrimental, and must therefore be eliminated, feel free to experiment with your meals. Enjoy new dishes, try out novel cooking ideas.

Have fun with your COUNTDOWN!

I have an interesting little anecdote here that will illustrate how most of us are simply not aware of what we eat. Anisa Ansari, one of my fitness class students, fell into this classic trap. Here is her story.

'One chapati is all I eat, but I'm still putting on weight doctor . . . '

Mrs Ansari's complaint was that in spite of eating very little, she kept putting on weight. When asked specifically by the physician, she replied, 'Only one chapati for lunch, and one for dinner.'

Her doctor probed further. He realized that Mrs Ansari was consuming much more than she thought she was. Through the day, she was having several high-calorie items that were not being accounted for.

He asked her to write down everything she consumed over the next twenty-four hours. Following his instructions, Mrs Ansari recorded her food intake through a typical day. The results were startling!

BREAKFAST

1. Bed tea—1 cup (half milk, half water)
2. 4 slices of bread, buttered

EVENING SNACK

1. 1 cold drink (300 ml)
2. 2 samosas

AFTER-DINNER SNACK

1. 1 gulab jamun
2. 1 soft drink (300 ml)

Without even taking lunch and dinner into account, Anisa Ansari was unwittingly consuming more calories than she had bargained for! Every deep-fried item she enjoyed added up to 35–40 per cent of pure fat. No wonder she was putting on weight.

Like Anisa, most of us probably feel we eat very little—'only one chapati for lunch and one for dinner'. But without realizing it, soft drinks, snacks on the run, farsan or biscuits with tea, all pile on the calories.

Food Item Substitute

Food Item	Substitute
Four slices of bread, buttered	Four slices of bread with a scraping of butter or mint chutney
Cold drink	Coconut water
Two samosas	Roasted savoury like kurmura bhel, khakra
Gulab jamun	One tablespoon dry fruit/chikki

It is therefore smart to do a reality check. Record your food intake on an average day and see where the extra calories are coming from. Is it the ghee on your rotis or the fried snacks at tea-time? Are you addicted to desserts or is cheese your big weakness?

Anisa was taught how to pick healthy, low-calorie foods that helped her lose weight. You too can do it.

The One-Day Recall is particularly important because, as you gradually ease yourself into the COUNTDOWN, it stops you from overindulging. You also discover, by experimenting, low-cal food options that you actually enjoy eating! Try to follow the One-Day Recall guidelines as faithfully as possible, to make the most of your FOUR-WEEK COUNTDOWN.

Please remember that the One-Day Recall is valid for the first three weeks of your diet only. From week four, your COUNTDOWN DIET becomes fully functional.

CHAPTER 5

SHOPPING & STOCKING

In this section I shall be going straight into your kitchen. To ensure your COUNTDOWN gets off to a great start, with no glitches and no 'oh-I've-run-out-of-XYZ-item', I recommend a written list of all the foods you need to stock. Save this list on your kitchen wall or on your desktop for easy reference.

Now, checklist in hand, let us run through your shelves to make sure you have all the must-haves—items you can't do without—at your fingertips.

Wholegrain cereals and pulses count as essentials. Buy whole grains and daal in bulk and store low-cal wholegrain snacks in your pantry. Make sure to keep the refrigerator stocked with fruits and veggies, or if you prefer, pick up your produce fresh every day. Milk and milk products are an all-important kitchen staple. If you are non-vegetarian, fill up your freezer with fish and poultry, in portion-sized packs for easy defrosting. Whenever stocks run low, check your list, and top up.

I am not for a moment suggesting that your kitchen be stocked with low-calorie items only. This is the real world. You have a family to feed, you have guests to entertain. In any case, the foods mentioned here are always great to have on hand, regardless of whether you are on a diet or not.

GREEN TIP

Greens like methi or lettuce leaves last longer if they are cleaned, dried, wrapped in kitchen-paper towels, then stored in plastic bags.

It's worth keeping in mind that being on a diet doesn't mean fried food should be out of bounds for everyone. What you can do is offer the higher calorie menus, in limited quantities, to guests and family. Cut your own allowance down to a bare minimum.

To give an example, let me tell you about one of my most successful clients, Steven Pinto. Rather than eat separate foods and feel like the odd one out, he ate whatever the family did. If there was moong dal, he would ask for the same thing, but without the ghee tadka. Or, if a cauliflower cheese bake was being made, he would tell his wife to take out his portion of steamed cauliflower before it went into the baking dish. Even for dessert, as the family devoured chocolate fudge brownies, he kept them company, with just half a piece.

If you have a cook at home, it is a good idea to inform them that you are going on a diet. One of my clients, Uma Iyer, made her life really simple by dedicating a couple of shelves in her kitchen cabinet to herself and storing all her diet ingredients there. So the cook knew exactly where to find her stuff. Cup and katori measures were also kept handy to further simplify things.

That's on the practical side. I have another client, Anita Shirodkar, who is more artistic. She loves colour. So she colour-codes her fruits and vegetables and makes sure every day of the week is different. On a purple day, Anita may have brinjals and figs, and use bajra as her cereal choice. On a yellow day, it could be moong dal, mosumbi and a pumpkin bake!

The point here is, your COUNTDOWN allows you the flexibility to choose. Be practical, be creative, be yourself.

Once your kitchen is well stocked, you can settle into the COUNTDOWN in no time at all. Use the ingredients as a source of inspiration to create your very own recipes and menus. Mix and match cuisines, be adventurous, learn to experiment. Try to introduce new tastes to keep your palate from getting jaded.

A word of advice here. Never go grocery shopping on an empty stomach, as you are always more tempted to pick up high-calorie foods, or munch something while you are ambling along the shopping aisles.

The list that follows covers the essential foods that you require for your COUNTDOWN. Please look out for the 'danger foods' list as well, and try to keep them at arm's length. Every time these foods come into your kitchen, beware!

STOCK UP	
Green/yellow moong daal	Onions
Brown rice	Apples
Broken wheat lapsi	Salad leaves
Bajre ka atta	Chaat masala
Jowar ka atta	Basil/oregano/rosemary

Whole-wheat bread	Green coriander and mint leaves
Multigrain bread	Lemons/limes
Rolled oats (oatmeal)	Green/herbal tea
Whole-wheat semolina (sooji)	Seasonal fruit
Whole-wheat crackers	Tomatoes/cucumber
Low-fat tofu	Leafy green vegetables
Low-fat paneer	Spices and herbs
Low-fat yoghurt	Apple cider vinegar
Skimmed milk	Balsamic vinegar
Low-fat feta cheese	Tomato puree

FOR NON-VEGETARIANS
Eggs
Lean fish/water-packed tuna
Chicken breast (white meat)
Shrimp

DIET NO-NOs	DIET OCCASIONALs
Ice cream	Potatoes
Deep-fried farsans	Bananas
Cakes and pastries	Peanut butter
Aerated soft drinks	Sweet potato
Potato wafers	Jackfruit
High-fat cheese	Mango
Mayonnaise	Chickoo
Jam/syrup	Sitaphal/Sharifa (custard apple)
Chocolates	
Desserts/puddings	

FOOD UNLIMITED		
Lime juice	Green chutney	Cloves
Chaat masala	Green chillis	Cardamom
Turmeric	Green coriander	Cinnamon
Chilli powder	Curry leaves	Pepper
Coriander powder	Mint leaves	Asafoetida

Jeera powder	Tamarind	Bay leaf
Sambar masala	Ginger	Nutmeg
Garam masala	Garlic	Kasuri methi

Q. I have heard tofu is very good for vegetarians. What is tofu and where can I get it?

A. Tofu is a soya bean product, produced by grinding cooked soya beans to make a milky substance that can then be solidified. It is also known as soya bean curd. Tofu is very high in protein and low in saturated fats. It is also cholesterol-free. A 100 gm serving of tofu contains around 73 calories. However, it is always a good idea to check the label. Firm tofu is low in fat, while softer tofu tends to have a higher fat content.

Tofu is naturally bland and makes an excellent paneer or cottage cheese substitute. Use it in sweet or savoury dishes. This product is stocked on supermarket shelves and in urban centres, small grocers will also carry the product.

Q. Can I have milk products?

A. Only low-fat or no-fat milk products are allowed. For example, buttermilk can be made with low-fat curds. Even paneer or cottage cheese can be made with low-fat milk and consumed in small quantities. High-fat milk products such as cheese, cream and butter should be avoided while on the COUNTDOWN.

Q. I love meat—can I have mutton regularly?

A. Mutton and pork are full of cholesterol and fat. You must steer clear of them during your COUNTDOWN. You could substitute meat with lean chicken or fish.

Q. Can I eat rice?

A. You can eat rice or any other cereal of your choice. However, it is essential that you stay within the recommended portion limit.

Q. Are vegetarian diets protein deficient?

A. No, vegetarians get their full supply of proteins from pulses and grains, milk and milk products and soya products. Animal sources such as milk and milk products are complete sources of protein. Vegetable proteins are incomplete and need to be combined with other foods. For example, grains and lentil (daal and chapati/rice), nuts or seeds with grains are excellent vegetarian protein sources.

The following list provides approximately the same amount of protein as 1 oz of meat (7 gm protein):

¼ cup cottage cheese or paneer
1 egg
½ cup legumes/lentil (cooked)
¼ cup tofu
1 cup soy milk
2 tablespoons mixed nuts

CHAPTER 6

MIND IT!

Prepare yourself mentally for the four weeks ahead

Did you know dieting is a mind game? Your brain is a very complex organ that has extremely complex responses. At a primal level, based on evolution, the brain wants you to retain body fat in case of drought or famine. It therefore has built-in checks and balances to prevent you from starving.

Modern society, however, has imposed a new set of rules for staying slim. Today, social pressures demand that you be svelte, if not actually skinny. The fashion industry promotes size-zero models. Film stars are constantly showing off super-toned bodies on screen. 'Yummy mummies' are the new super moms who get back their pre-pregnancy figures in no time at all. Even middle-aged men, well into their forties, maintain their abs, build up their muscles, and end up looking half their age.

So what are we missing here? Why do overweight people put on weight in the first place?

You have probably heard the saying, 'You can't be too thin or too rich!' Today, millions of like-minded people all over the world actually work very hard at being slim. They build their lives around maintaining their weight and staying healthy. How do they do it?

They do not give in to temptation. More important, they do not give up.

While this may seem obvious, please pause and give it a serious thought. I have just said something very very crucial. Your mind influences all your actions. So, if you make a conscious decision to stop overeating, your body has no choice but to obey! If you do make the occasional mistake, like we all do from time to time, your willpower will see you through. But if your resolve weakens, and you fail to control a passing urge to binge, your weight loss attempts will go nowhere.

The brain deals with stress in different ways. In rare cases, the pressure to be thin is so overwhelming that it leads to unnatural eating disorders, like anorexia nervosa. This is a condition where a switch in your brain makes you go into starvation mode and it requires medical intervention. I will not go into the details about the causes of such problems here—I simply want to emphasize that as far as your diet is concerned, it's mind over matter. Every time.

So start by making a pact with yourself. Write down your intention, specify how much weight you want to lose. Or tell someone you trust, a supportive friend or spouse, about your weight loss goals. Many dieters go public with their weight problem and this can be a very powerful motivator. For then it no longer remains a private commitment and it makes you accountable to somebody else other than yourself.

I have compiled a little quiz to help you understand how your mind works and what your weaknesses might be. Please try to answer as honestly as possible!

QUICK QUIZ

How to think thin

Read the ten statements, think carefully, then answer with a clear 'Yes' or 'No'.

YES OR NO

1. I follow strict diets and give up after a few days.
2. I have no time to eat frequently.
3. I am too busy to exercise.
4. I can't resist temptation.
5. I stress eat most of the time.
6. I don't like the way I look.
7. Low-calorie foods are so uninteresting.
8. I can't control my appetite.
9. I eat when I am bored.
10. I feel bad to say 'no' to anything I am served when I am invited out.

If you've answered 'No' to at least seven of them, consider yourself a positive dieter. You recognize your diet pitfalls and are able to work towards maintaining self-discipline. You are on your way to feeling fit, fab and in control.

If seven or more questions have a 'Yes' answer, you have work to do. Don't worry, the following section specifically identifies and addresses your weak spots, and helps you to work towards result-oriented solutions.

MAKE A FRESH START

It's time to review your mindset and lifestyle. Very often, the make-or-break point is a split-second decision. If you understand the circumstances that lead to diet mistakes, and the consequences of making those mistakes, chances are you will be more aware.

This is not going to be easy. Like I mentioned earlier, you are genetically hard-wired to eat, so resisting food goes against your grain and against your natural instincts. But always tell yourself, you can do it. Keep going back to your X factor, your reason for wanting to lose weight.

Why did you decide to diet? What is the reward you are looking for? Every time you pick up a fried snack, ask yourself, is this going to get me my reward? Is it worth sacrificing my diet for the momentary pleasure of eating this? Or can I satiate my craving with a piece of fruit?

NOTHING SUCCEEDS LIKE SUCCESS

If you can put that fried snack down and turn your head away, you have won a major victory! It's a bit like winning a match, or securing a plum job. The more you succeed, the more confident you become. And the more confident you get, the more likely you are to achieve your goals.

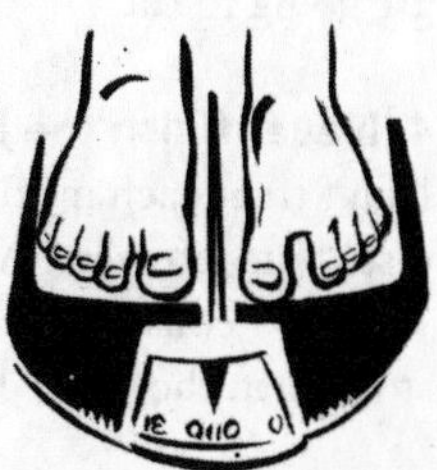

TEN TIPS TO TIP THE SCALES IN YOUR FAVOUR

1. Think thin

Think yourself thin and automatically you are channeling your energies in a positive direction. This has the most amazing results! When you think positive, you attain your goal in a single-minded, focused manner.

Remember, it's all about the feel good factor. Even if you go off track occasionally, do not be consumed by guilt. Never say, 'I've started to exercise, but so far I have lost only two pounds'; instead say, 'I feel great after losing two pounds, now I am inspired to continue exercising.'

2. Don't stress about being fat

Did you know, if you worry about being fat, you will be. Stress can lead to emotional eating, a factor that contributes to weight gain. There is a tendency to go for 'comfort foods', such as sweets or fried snacks and very often, the amount consumed goes up as well. This double whammy takes its toll and ultimately, shows up on your weighing scale.

3. Make your meals attractive and appetizing

Visual appeal enhances the flavour of your food! When you see an attractive presentation, a beautifully arranged table, multi-hued salad veggies, cut in an unusual way, colourfully garnished dishes, with toppings such as coriander, you feel good about the food you are going to eat.

4. Never finish the leftovers

Don't treat each meal as if it is your last supper. Refrigerate or distribute leftovers. Ask naturally slim people what they eat and you will get a consistent answer. They eat when they are hungry and stop when they have had enough.

5. When tempted to indulge, go brush your teeth

When you are about to give in to temptation, go brush your teeth. Not only does this work wonders, your craving will have passed!

6. Never go grocery shopping on an empty stomach

The surest way of sabotaging your diet is to go to the supermarket when you are hungry. On an empty stomach, you are more likely to fill up your trolley with indulgences you would not otherwise pick! So make sure you eat something before setting out.

7. Learn the art of savouring food

When you eat slowly, you savour your food and relish your meal. This not only helps to digest food better, but also prevents overeating.

8. Make smart food choices

Eat nutritious food. Make wholesome choices, avoid packaged, refined foods. Be creative in preparing tasty, low-cal meals that you will really enjoy.

9. Think before you drink

When you drink, understand that you are consuming empty calories. If you wish to drink occasionally, follow the guidelines given in the Drinking & Dieting chapter.

10. Hydrate yourself

Drink at least eight glasses of water a day. Also eat high water content foods that will help you lose weight. Examples are watermelon, oranges, pineapples, tomatoes and cucumber.

CHAPTER 7

FAT MAKES YOU FAT

Regardless of what anyone tells you, remember this: Fat makes you fat. It is as simple as that. Fat is loaded with calories and you can only lose weight if your calorie 'input', which is your food consumption, is *less than* your calorie 'output', which is the calories you burn off through the day.

I know how hard it is to cut out the fried stuff. In a weak moment, that jalebi looks like it's begging to be consumed. Or a pack of chips seems like the answer to life's problems. Believe me, it is simply not worth it. Tell yourself you could consume a delicious, sweet, juicy fruit, and be just as happy. Well, almost.

Whenever you pass up the puri for the roti, congratulate yourself. Once you make the initial effort, you will find it gets easier to spurn the samosas and ditch the desserts. But don't just stop there. Go gift yourself a trendy accessory. Try out a new perfume. These little things work as huge morale boosters because, not only did you say no to fat, you did something special for yourself.

As we go further into this chapter, you will understand why an excessive fat intake can wreak havoc on your diet!

One gram of fat equals nine calories. One gram of carbohydrate or one gram of protein equals four calories.

As you can see, compared to proteins and carbohydrates, fats contain more than double the calories; so it is obvious why dieters must severely restrict their fat intake. Limiting fat in your diet automatically brings down the overall calorie consumption.

Visible fats such as oil, butter, ghee and margarine can be easily identified. But there are hidden fats present in almost all foods, in varying amounts. For example, cheese could have milk fat of up to 70 per cent. Oily fish such as tuna or sardine also have a high fat content. Even certain vegetables, like avocado or olive, are high in fat.

While some amount of fat is required in your diet, it has to be kept to a minimum. In fact, dieters should cut their fat consumption to roughly 10 per cent of their daily calorie intake.

What happens when supply exceeds demand?

If you put extra petrol in a car with a full tank, the tank overflows. In the same way, if your body has a daily requirement of, let's say 1700 calories, but you insist on stuffing yourself with 2000 calories, the extra 300 calories 'overflow'.

This overflow turns into fat and gets stored in your fat cells. If more and more fat keeps coming in, the cells are forced to expand. There comes a point when the cells expand so much that they can no longer store the excess fat, so they multiply to make room for all the additional fat that is coming in.

When fat intake is reduced, fat cells shrink in size, but never disappear. So once fat cells have been formed, the number of fat cells does not decrease.

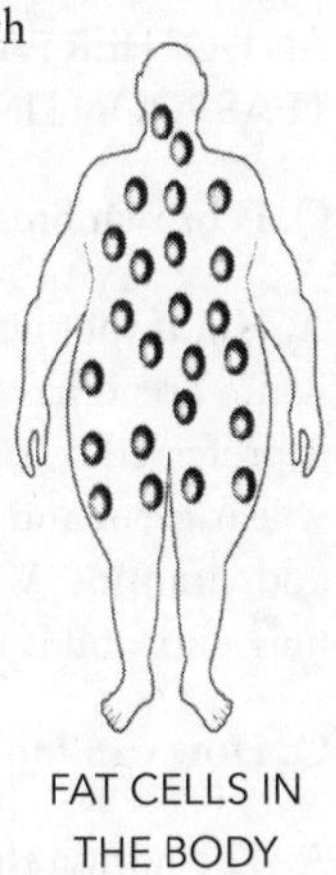

FAT CELLS IN THE BODY

Q. Are all types of oils and fats equal as far as calories are concerned?

A. Yes. Every type of oil—groundnut, sunflower, mustard, olive, sesame or any other—contain nine calories per gram. Butter and ghee also add up to nine calories per gram. If you want to lose weight, it is crucial to limit your daily consumption of fats to a maximum of two teaspoons.

Q. What are good fats and bad fats? What does it mean?

A. Examples of good fats are monounsaturated fats such as olive, peanut and canola oil. Polyunsaturated fats, from plant sources such as corn and sunflower, are also considered beneficial. These are considered good fats because, when consumed in small quantities, they reduce the cholesterol in blood and protect against heart diseases.

However, ayurveda encourages the consumption of ghee. In India, traditional cooking methods make use of ghee, butter and locally available cooking oil. So, while there is a case for choosing monounsaturated and polyunsaturated fats, during your COUNTDOWN, butter and ghee are also perfectly acceptable.

THE BOTTOM LINE: CHOOSE GHEE, BUTTER, OLIVE OIL OR ANY OTHER FAT AS LONG AS YOU STAY WITHIN YOUR TWO TEASPOON LIMIT!

Q. Is brown bread less fattening than white bread?

A. No, if the slice of bread is the same size, brown bread and white bread have equal calorific value. The reason brown bread is preferred by dieticians is because it is unrefined food, with the wheat germ and husk intact, thereby making it a rich source of fibre and vitamins. White bread, on the other hand, has been stripped of nutrients and is refined, or is 'empty' calories.

Q. How can food be tasty without adding oil?

A. The notion that oil adds to taste is a misconception. You can fry your masalas in oil, and it is the masalas that add flavour to your food, not the oil! Vegetables and daals have their own unique taste and this can be enhanced with zero-calorie masalas, herbs and condiments, without using a drop of oil.

FACT FILE

One chapati contains ninety calories. A large spoonful of ghee spread over the chapati doubles the calorie count, to 180 calories!

The ghee on your chapati, the butter on your bread, and the oil in your cooking—what is the best way to reduce them all? See how you can cook great-tasting Indian food without the use of fat, yet your dish will be delicious!

FAT-FREE ZERO-OIL COUNTDOWN MASALA

1. Heat a kadai or non-stick pan.
2. Roast cumin seeds (jeera) until they crackle and turn light brown.
3. Add chopped onion and keep stirring. If the onion starts sticking to the sides, add a few drops of water, and continue stirring.
4. Add ginger and garlic paste to your taste. Roast this masala paste to a light brown. Avoid adding more water, as too much water will give the masala a boiled taste.
5. Add tomato paste and once again, blend in with a minimum amount of water.
6. Now add all the other powdered masalas—turmeric, red chilli powder, coriander powder and garam masala to taste.
7. Roast all ingredients together until a great aroma wafts up.

Your basic COUNTDOWN MASALA is ready! Use this for all your vegetable and daal preparations and, as you keep experimenting, you can introduce variations in the masala. When your dish is ready, garnish it with chopped green coriander, green chillis, chaat masala and lime juice, to suit your taste.

NON-STICK COOKWARE

Try to use non-stick pans and utensils for cooking. For instance, a vegetable made in a non-stick pan can be made with a few drops of oil. The same vegetable would burn or stick in a regular utensil.

FOUR-WEEK COUNTDOWN ROADMAP
Your Diet Diary

UPSIDE	DOWNSIDE
WEEK 1 enthusiasm for new plan **only one diet meal**	adjustment phase **self-control over other meals** not feeling completely full
WEEK 2 **Hearty, healthy breakfast** high morning energy level	**breakfast skippers must find time** temptation to snack indiscriminately **sense of deprivation**
WEEK 3 frequent snacking **feeling of well-being** signs of weight loss	planning your snacks properly **diet resolve weakening** occasional cheating bouts
WEEK 4 **full plan kicks in** end in sight **scale shows results**	**desire to binge** wanting to give up in weak moments **unrealistic fourth week expectations**

CHAPTER 8

COUNTDOWN DINNER

Wind down your day, cut down your dinner

Dinner is the first COUNTDOWN meal you must modify. Many of you may ask: why is it necessary to cut down on dinner first? There is a very good reason for it.

Why cut down on dinner first?

The fact is, this is the time of the day when your physical activity is tapering off. You are tired, your energy levels are probably dropping. This makes you extremely vulnerable. Your natural instinct is to grab all the 'comfort foods' you can lay your hands on.

For some of you, your social life begins after sunset. You might start with a drink at the club. Or you may dine out at a restaurant. Many of you may attend family functions, where food is the highlight of the evening. So how do you resist all the temptation coming your way? While it is not easy, controlling binge-eating at dinner-time is a key factor in weight loss.

Consider this simple proposition. If you overindulge at dinner-time and sleep on a full stomach, the excess calories you consume have nowhere to go, and will most likely end up around your waistline. This is because, during the night, your body goes into rest mode. When you fall asleep, you cannot burn off all the excess calories that you have consumed, so this surplus energy gets stored as fat.

Surely it does not require a genius to figure this all out! Cutting down on dinner is therefore a crucial first step towards weight loss.

SEVEN DAYS TO FORM A HABIT

It is a scientifically proven fact that it takes seven days for human beings to accept any change in their routine. After seven days, the new variant becomes a habit. Keeping this in mind, I have used seven-day cycles to introduce changes in your FOUR-WEEK COUNTDOWN, giving you time to adjust to your diet on a week-by-week basis.

For me personally, calorie-watching at dinner-time is like seeing a great movie but missing out on the ending! Or getting to a really fabulous beach destination, only to find it raining!

If you feel dinner is the most difficult meal to cut back on, you have my full sympathy. I feel exactly the same way. Coming from a large Indian family, dinner had always been a family food-fest. My mother, a fabulous cook, painstakingly catered to our love for good food and, as a result, dinners were always spectacular.

The cuisine varied every day and we kept thinking of new ways to tease our palates. Continental. Indian. Thai. Spanish. Italian.

Morrocan. You name it and we were ready to savour the next culinary experience from exotic destinations around the world, discovering unique new flavours, devouring every last morsel!

Then there was the added attraction of family members coming together, bonding after a hard day at work. After all, who doesn't enjoy the prospect of getting home to a nice, hearty dinner? Along with great company and great conversation, dinner was a special occasion every day.

But this was precisely the problem. Inevitably, slowly but surely, the kilos started piling up. We couldn't continue to eat as we did and still keep our weight under control. Something had to give. Earlier, while planning dinner menus, the last thing on our minds was calorie restriction. So it had to be a conscious decision. The effort was to make food enjoyable, without going overboard on the calories.

Even today my mother gets out the most amazing food on the table. But we stay away from buttery sauces and creamy gravies. We still eat delicious food and we still drool over every bite. The menus are just as tasty but everything is lighter and more balanced. And yes, I'd like to add, the conversation continues to be as lively as ever.

FOUR-COURSE BALANCED DINNER PLAN

Your FOUR-WEEK COUNTDOWN dinner is certainly about controlling portions and cutting excess fat, but you can hardly complain about feeling deprived! In fact, your dinner packs in tons of nutrition, as every bite is loaded with vitamins and minerals, proteins and carbs, and the recommended allowance of fats.

I earnestly request you to follow the diet as closely as possible, to get the best results. Remember, what you put in is what you will get out.

During your FOUR-WEEK COUNTDOWN dinner, please remember to eat regularly, preferably no later than 9 p.m. (so that you don't sleep on a full stomach). Do not eat more than the prescribed portions, but do not skip any courses either. Even if you feel full after the third course, it is essential to complete the entire dinner plan. This helps you avoid a midnight trip to the refrigerator, which is the last thing you want to do!

The idea is to feel satisfied, not stuffed, after you finish your four course dinner plan.

LIQUIDS, MORE LIQUIDS, SOLIDS, AND A LITTLE BIT OF EMPTY SPACE

During dinner, you will be filling yourself with a liquid, then another slightly thicker liquid, followed by a portion of fibre, which works as a high water-content appetizer, and lastly, a main course. While the quality and quantity of your food is important, it is equally important to leave a little bit of space in your stomach empty. This allows the digestive juices to do their work efficiently.

¼ liquids ½ solids ¼ empty

The initial consumption of liquids and fibre helps to quench your hunger pangs, so by the time you get to the main course, you are already beginning to feel full. This way it becomes easier to stay within the limits of the portion-controlled main course menu. Initially, you may find the extra liquid intake hard to handle but in a week's time, you should settle down.

> Contrary to popular belief, water does not dilute digestive juices.
>
> Eat at least two hours before sleeping

DINNER FORMULA

1. Starter Sips
2. Nutri Bowl

3. Fibre Filler
4. Main Course as per diet plan—Plan Minimum/Plan Medium/ Plan Maximum

Remember, before you start your main course dinner, there are three mini courses you have to consume—Starter Sips, Nutri Bowl and Fibre Filler. These work as nutrition boosters and keep you feeling full.

UNLIMITED STARTER SIPS

Keep in mind that the STARTER SIPS are basically a negligible calorie, 'drink as much as you want', start to your meal. They consist of an unlimited amount of light, watery liquids to start you off. You gently whet your appetite by introducing an easy-to-digest liquid as your first course. It works as an initial filler and also aids digestion. Your stomach begins to get into gear.

STARTER SIPS (unlimited)

coconut water
or
clear soup—clear part of vegetable stock
or
herbal tea—green, cinnamon, mint, ginger, chamomile or jasmine
or
fresh lime juice (salted)
or
moong water
or
rasam
or
jeera pani
or
chicken bullion soup

Check out STARTER SIPS RECIPES at the end of this chapter.

NUTRI BOWL 2 katoris (1 cup)

After you sip, you slurp! The NUTRI BOWL is a more substantial course, to be consumed within the recommended serving allowance. This course is a more robust liquid, in the form of a soup (without cereals such as noodles, rice or pasta), veggie juice or low-cal buttermilk. It is heavier than the first course, and is a perfect follow up to the digestive liquid. All your NUTRI BOWL options come loaded with combinations of vitamins, minerals and proteins, and practically no fat. Varying NUTRI BOWL choices on a daily basis gives you delicious variations.

FACT FILE

Research shows that people who consume soup before starting on their main meal consume about a hundred calories less than those who omit the soup course. People who watch their weight have also consistently recorded that soup has helped tremendously in their diet plans.

NUTRI BOWL 2 katoris (1 cup)

soup—hot or cold
or
vegetable juice
or

buttermilk—use ½ katori (¼ cup) skimmed curd
or
thin kadhi—use ½ katori (¼ cup) skimmed curd
or
egg drop soup

Check out NUTRI BOWL RECIPES at the end of this chapter.

FIBRE FILLER 2 katoris (1 cup)

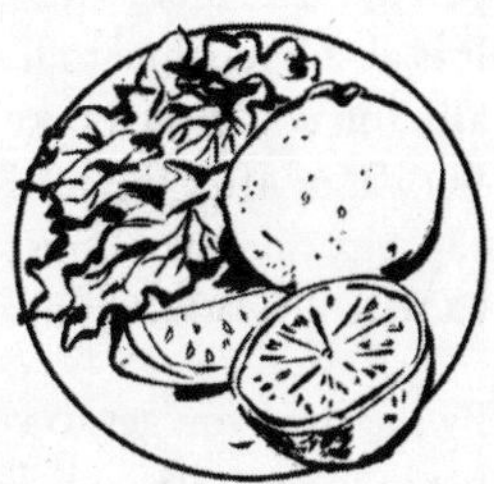

Your third course, the FIBRE FILLER, puts you onto a fibre-rich, moisture-rich filler. Think juicy veggies, fruits, crisp sprouts, crunchy salads and you get the idea. The FIBRE FILLER must be chewed slowly and thoroughly, because the digestion process begins in your mouth itself.

This helps you properly absorb the valuable nutrients that are so good for you. Moreover, when you eat slowly, you feel like you are eating more, plus you give your taste buds full enjoyment!

Another bonus is that your FIBRE FILLER has very limited calories, making it a guilt-free munch and crunch. A dash of lime juice, chaat masala, a bit of rock salt and pepper add extra zest to your FIBRE FILLER options. Take a look at some of the choices you have.

FIBRE FILLER 2 katoris (1 cup)

2 katoris (1 cup) veggie salad—tomato, cucumber, carrot, celery, lettuce
or
2 katoris (1 cup) fruit salad—orange, apple, sweet lime, pear, papaya
or

2 katoris (1 cup) fruit and veggie salad—apple, celery, lettuce, sweet lime

Check out FIBRE FILLER RECIPES at the end of this chapter.

ARRIVING AT THE MAIN COURSE

Many of you may not be used to consuming such high volumes of liquids or crunching through so much fibre! If all this really fills you up, take a breather before getting onto the MAIN COURSE. It is absolutely fine to have a gap between courses, no problem at all. You could even take a break after the STARTER SIP or NUTRI BOWL or after the FIBRE FILLER. Work the gaps as per your capacity and take time to savour every bit of your four-course COUNTDOWN dinner!

By the time you get to your MAIN COURSE, you will already begin to feel satisfied. This helps you to stay within the requirements of your diet dinner without a sense of being deprived. Follow the MAIN COURSE according to the plan you are slotted into—**Plan Minimum, Plan Medium** or **Plan Maximum.**

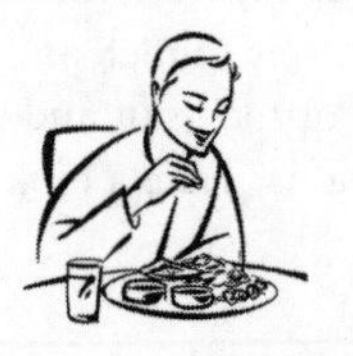

MAIN COURSE DINNER

Your COUNTDOWN Dinner Main Course is divided into three distinct food groups:

1. CEREALS
2. FRUITS AND VEGETABLES
3. PROTEIN RICH FOODS

What could be simpler than remembering 1, 2, 3?

At any point in your COUNTDOWN, you know the menu is not complete unless you count 1, 2, 3! It's your way of making sure that the three food groups are always included. You could be dining at home, eating out, on the go, among friends, alone, it does not matter, as long as your meals add up to 1, 2, 3.

Consider the 1, 2, 3 Formula to be your diet staple for all meals. 1 is for cereal, your energy provider. 2 represents fruits and vegetables, for your supply of vitamins and minerals. And 3 stands for protein-rich foods, to look after repair and re-growth of body tissue. I have devised the 1, 2, 3 Formula as a means of ensuring balanced nutrition for every single COUNTDOWN meal that you consume.

Apart from the 1, 2, 3 Formula, there is one more important component. You are allowed ½ a teaspoon of any fat with your dinner. It could be cooking oil, butter, cream or ghee, the choice is yours.

You may wonder why 1, 2, 3 Formula is such a big deal. Look around you. Observe people who are on a crash diet. Do you see dark circles or dull skin? Do you hear complaints about falling hair, or feeling listless? With the COUNTDOWN, you will have no such problems. All thanks to 1, 2, 3!

REMINDER

Choose your dinner MAIN COURSE based on how much weight you need to lose. Please refer to my Plan Minimum, Plan Medium and Plan Maximum to slot yourself correctly.

Also check your Daily Food Guide in Annexure B to understand 'What makes one serving?' This determines the serving size of cereals, fruit and veggies and protein-rich foods allowed for your particular Plan.

A quick reference table is provided here. For clarifications and more options, please refer to Annexure B.

PLAN MINIMUM Dinner

for women to lose up to four kilos

DINNER FORMULA

1. Starter Sips: unlimited
2. Nutri Bowl: 2 katoris (1 cup)
3. Fibre Filler: 2 katoris (1 cup)
4. 1, 2, 3 Main Course as given below:

1 CEREALS ½ serving

1 small phulka or 1 small slice of bread (made of any cereal)
or
½ katori cooked cereal of your choice (rice, pasta, poha, rawa)

+

2 FRUIT & VEGETABLES 1 serving

1 katori of your choice (restrict potato, jackfruit, yam, banana)

+

3 PROTEIN-RICH FOODS 1 serving

1 katori moong dal or sprouts
or
4 cubes low-fat paneer/feta cheese/tofu/1 katori low-fat curd
or
1 medium-sized piece white meat (chicken/turkey breast or fish)
or
2 egg whites

PLAN MEDIUM dinner

for men to lose up to 4 kilos or for women to lose 5–10 kilos

DINNER FORMULA

1. Starter Sips: unlimited
2. Nutri Bowl: 2 katoris (1 cup)
3. Fibre Filler: 2 katoris (1 cup)
4. 1, 2, 3 Main Course as given below:

1 CEREALS 1 serving

2 small phulkas/1 large roti/1 large slice of bread (made of any cereal)
or
1 katori cooked cereal of your choice (rice, pasta, poha, rawa)

\+

2 FRUIT & VEGETABLES 1 serving

1 katori of your choice (restrict potato, jackfruit, yam, banana, mango)

\+

3 PROTEIN-RICH FOODS 1 serving

1 katori moong dal or sprouts
or
4 cubes low-fat paneer/feta cheese/tofu/1 katori low-fat curd
or
1 medium-sized piece white meat (chicken/turkey breast or fish)
or
2 egg whites

PLAN MAXIMUM dinner

for men to lose more than 5 kilos or for women to lose more than 11 kilos

DINNER FORMULA

1. Starter Sips: unlimited
2. Nutri Bowl: 2 katoris (1 cup)
3. Fibre Filler: 2 katoris (1 cup)
4. 1, 2, 3 Main Course as given below:

1 CEREAL 1 serving

2 small phulkas/1 large roti/1 large slice of bread (made of any cereal)
or
1 katori cooked cereal of your choice (rice, pasta, poha, rawa)

+

2 FRUIT & VEGETABLES 1 serving

1 katori of your choice (restrict potato, jackfruit, yam, banana)

+

3 PROTEIN-RICH FOODS 2 servings

2 katoris moong dal or sprouts
or
8 cubes low-fat paneer/feta cheese/tofu/2 katoris low-fat curd
or
2 medium-sized piece white meat (chicken/turkey breast or fish)
or
4 egg whites

WHAT IF YOU ARE STILL HUNGRY?

Initially, you might find it difficult to stay within the prescribed portions. If you feel hungry after your Main Course, you can have one more helping of the NUTRI BOWL or FIBRE FILLER. If you are still not satisfied, have one more portion of either option. This is better than consuming extra cereal during your meal, because cereals are high in carbohydrates. Another important tip: Avoid lingering at the dining table when you have finished your meal, as you may end up munching unnecessarily.

Please do remember: being slightly hungry is normal! Your stomach should remain ¼ empty to aid digestion, and in a few days, you'll get used to the lighter dinners.

FACT FILE

Your stomach is like a balloon. As you eat less food, your stomach starts shrinking within 3 to 4 weeks of your diet. You automatically eat less, because you tend to feel full more quickly.

POST-DINNER SOS

Ideally, dinner should be consumed at least two hours before bed-time. This sometimes leads to a craving for a 'bed-time snack'. While the COUNTDOWN does not permit snacking before sleeping—it will spell doom for your diet—I have included some options that will satisfy the urge to munch something. Please understand these are by no means snack substitutes, but merely a means of satisfying the sensory requirement for that late night snack!

Cardamom, cinnamon sticks, saunf (aniseed), sugarless gum, even some herbal tea are some of the SOS options you can try. The comfort of chewing or drinking will settle you down and, in fact, most of these options are great digestive aids as well.

DINNER VARIATIONS

3-in-1 Dinner

Stay with Starter Sips, then combine the rest of your meal

On evenings when you are pressed for time, you can opt for a One-dish Dinner. This option allows you begin with your STARTER SIPS, in unlimited quantities, followed by a combination of the 3 remaining courses—your NUTRI BOWL, FIBRE FILLER and Main Course.

The quantities for all items remain exactly the same as the 4-course COUNTDOWN dinner; the only difference is that you combine the courses in a delicious one-dish meal.

Check out the 3-in-1 Dinner RECIPES at the end of this chapter.

DINING OUT

To all you party animals out there, I have to emphasize that the success of your diet depends largely on restricting dinners out. However, there will be times when you find yourself socializing in the evening, eating out at a restaurant, or having a meal with friends and family. Keep dining out to a minimum. This is because you have little control over the menu and are often tempted to binge when you see others around you doing the same.

If you have to be out at a restaurant, order judiciously. Please refer to what you can eat before you step out. Remember the thumb rule: no deep fried foods, no desserts, no aerated soft drinks. Opt for steamed and lightly sautéed dishes without heavy sauces and gravies.

Tip: When you are done with your dinner, ask for your plate to be cleared. Otherwise, you may end up eating mindlessly, just because the food is in front of you.

Time and again, I have reiterated that the COUNTDOWN works around you and your lifestyle. For those of you who end up partying late into the night, I have devised a plan that can help you eat right even as you enjoy your social life! Have a 'part dinner' at home, before you leave for your party. You could consume your STARTER SIPS and NUTRI BOWL at home, then proceed with your Main Course Dinner at the party. This way you are not ravenous at dinner-time, and are able to stick to controlled portions.

THE CASE OF THE HUNGRY HOUSEWIFE

A friend of mine, Rekha Kale, came to me desperate for advice. Rekha had tried all kinds of diet dinners—the soup and salad diet, the high protein diet, the low-carb diet, the no-carb diet and, in desperation, even starved! But not only did she fail to cut down on her food, she ended up eating a lot more. Not just that, she felt ravenous again in just an hour!

What is the best course for Rekha?

Rekha was trying to lose weight without listening to her body. She simply had to go back to the basics. Any diet plan that advocates the elimination of certain food groups, or restricts essential nutrients, is bound to deprive the body of a balanced diet.

And the body is going to respond by craving the food it needs.

I asked Rekha to sit down and first of all take a deep breath. I explained the importance of catering to her body's needs. She required a menu that covered all the essential food groups, in the right quantities. This included cereals for energy, fruit and vegetables for vitamins and minerals, and protein-rich foods for repair and growth of body tissue.

Rekha had been avoiding cereals in her diet and therefore craved quick-acting refined carbs such as candy and chocolates, which caused a rapid rise in her blood sugar and serotonin levels. This promoted a feeling of well-being for a brief period, followed by a sudden drop in energy levels.

It was therefore vital for her to reintroduce cereals into her diet plan again. The cereal intake would automatically reduce her carbohydrate cravings, because her body would no longer demand chocolates as a quick fix to raise her blood sugar level. Instead, a steady supply of complex carbs in her diet would provide the substance and roughage needed to keep her feeling full through the night.

Rekha followed the plan diligently. Instead of staying awake fighting hunger pangs, she managed to sleep through the night. The real reward? Rekha shed her excess weight over 6 months and, by maintaining her sensible eating habits, has kept it off.

THE CASE OF THE BLOATING BANKER

Another interesting case is that of Mishra Uncle. An old friend of my father's, Mishra Uncle is a busy man who is out at business dinners several days in a month. He was fed up with the late dinners and the rich restaurant food. They left him feeling bloated and uncomfortable all night. This 'conspicuous consumption' also added inches to his waistline.

How could Mishra Uncle help himself ?

By recognizing he had a problem, Mishra Uncle had already taken the first step towards rectifying the situation. I invited him for a home-cooked dinner, and along with the roti-sabzi, offered him some practical advice.

All he had to do was follow a 4-course dinner plan whenever he ate out. Starting with a herbal tea to aid digestion, Mishra Uncle could move on to a cup of veggie soup followed by a crunchy salad and then a balanced main course.

Sometimes, he felt hungry even after the main course. I allowed him an extra helping of salad, with some chaat masala and lemon.

Over time, Mishra Uncle was able to follow his new regimen with ease. At the same time, he could keep his business colleagues company, course after course. At the end of the meal, he felt well-satisfied, without being stuffed. His stomach always remained ¼ empty, important for minimizing bloating and discomfort.

His waistline shrunk and Mishra Uncle was grateful and blessed me for my advice. I would also like to add here—he blamed me too, for having to spend on a new wardrobe!

In the context of dinner, some common questions pop up all the time. My clients come with all sorts of queries—some valid, and some with no basis whatsoever. Here are the answers to some frequently asked questions.

Q. I have heard you mustn't have carbs at night—is this true?

A. No, this is a myth. It might surprise you to know that most of the food you eat contains carbs. Milk, cereals, vegetables, fruit, pulses—all these foods contain carbs in varying proportions. Only meat, fish and eggs are carb-free. It is essential to maintain a balanced diet that includes carbs and proteins—in fact, carbs should make up 55–60 per cent of your diet, as they are the body's main source of energy.

Only if you consume carbohydrates in excess will the surplus be stored as fat. An inadequate supply of carbs could lead to low blood sugar levels, known as hypoglycemia.

Compare calories of carbs or proteins to fat calories:

1 g carbs/1 g protein = 4 cal per g
1 g fat = 9 cal per g

DID YOU KNOW?

Fruit and vegetables are examples of carbohydrate-rich foods that have great nutritional value, as they are loaded with fibre, essential vitamins and minerals.

Q. To lose weight, should I stop eating after 7 p.m.?

A. If you stop eating after 7 p.m., you will be hungry by 10 p.m.! This is a highly impractical diet plan, as most people commute back from work during this hour and cannot be expected to focus on dinner.

After dinner, it is advisable to maintain a gap of two hours before bedtime, so that you avoid sleeping on a full stomach. There will be times when you end up eating a late dinner, but this is a minor glitch. Just make sure you stick with your COUNTDOWN diet and keep going.

REMINDERS TO PASTE ON THE REFRIGERATOR

1. Brush your teeth straight after dinner, then you are not tempted to snack.
2. Affirmation before dinner: 'I will succeed with this diet plan; I have the determination to succeed'.
3. Write down your motivation to lose weight in red ink, and as a reminder keep that paper pasted or hung in a place where you can see it.
4. Find an interesting after-dinner activity to keep your mind off food. (Chess with the children, Facebook time on the Net!)
5. If you feel so hungry that you can't sleep, pick one option from the SOS section. Repeat affirmation.
6. Put up a sign on your refrigerator: CLOSED AFTER DINNER
7. If you haven't had at least six glasses of water through the day, now is the time to top up.
8. Don't succumb to temptation from well-meaning family and friends who say, 'But you have to eat, it's my birthday!', or 'Come on, one puri won't do any harm!' Believe me, it will.
9. Never snack while watching your favourite late-night show.
10. Keep your SOS snack handy, just in case.

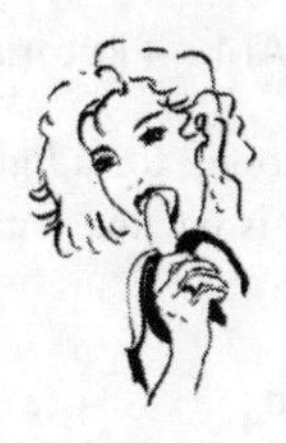

DINNER RECIPES

1 katori = ½ cup = 100 ml
2 katoris = 1 cup = 200 ml

STARTER SIP RECIPES

Allowance = unlimited

CHICKEN BULLION SOUP 8 katoris (4 cups)

A light chicken stock soup with its own subtle flavour.

Ingredients

1 medium-sized broiler chicken	8 katoris water
3–4 bay leaves	Salt to taste
2–3 pods garlic	Lime wedges (optional)

Method

Wash the broiler and remove skin completely. Boil in pressure cooker or pan, with 4 cups of water, bay leaves, garlic and salt to taste. Cook until meat comes off the bone. Once it is cooked, remove the chicken from the bullion soup. Strain the clear broth, adjust seasoning. When you are having the bullion soup, you can squeeze a few drops of fresh lime juice for extra flavour.

NOTE: De-bone the chicken and use it for chicken salad, baked dishes, with pasta, or in a sandwich with mustard.

MODIFIED TOMATO RASAM 4 katoris (2 cups)

Substitute tuvar dal with moong for a lighter rasam. This version tastes almost the same, and is packed with zingy flavours!

Ingredients

4 katoris water from cooked moong dal
2 teaspoons rasam powder
2 large ripe tomatoes
¼ teaspoon urad dal (optional)
handful curry leaves
pinch of asafoetida (hing)
bunch of fresh coriander leaves

Method

Skim off the clear water from the top of the cooked moong dal to make 4 katoris of liquid. Skin and cut the tomatoes into large chunks and add to the daal-water mixture. Put the mixture to boil in a saucepan. Stir in rasam masala.

Once the tomatoes soften, temper with urad dal, curry leaves and asafoetida. (You can do a dry tempering—ghee or oil not required.) Garnish with chopped coriander leaves. Serve piping hot.

PUDINA JEERA PAANI 8 katoris (4 cups)

In the mood for something tangy? This pungent drink really hits the spot.

Ingredients

8 katoris water
4 teaspoons tamarind pulp
4 teaspoons fresh lime juice
1 teaspoon fresh ginger paste
1 teaspoon roasted, ground cumin
½ teaspoon rock salt (kala namak)
2–3 sprigs fresh mint leaves (garnish)

Method

Mix the tamarind pulp extract and all the above ingredients, except the mint leaves, into the water. Stir well. Refrigerate for 2 hours, then strain through a fine sieve. Add finely chopped mint leaves. Drink chilled, with ice if desired.

MOONG WATER 8 katoris (4 cups)

A very lightly flavoured liquid with a nutty moong taste. You can omit the turmeric, or substitute it with cumin powder if desired.

Ingredients

2 katoris whole green moong dal
8 katoris water
pinch turmeric
salt to taste

Method

Boil the moong dal with turmeric and salt in a pressure cooker. When it is cooked, ladle off the clear water from the top. Drink this slightly warm (the rest of the daal can be used for dinner recipes).

MINT & BASIL TEA 4 katoris (2 cups)

A great decoction to soothe your throat and settle your tummy!

Ingredients

1–2 sprigs mint leaves
1–2 sprigs Indian basil leaves (tulsi)
8 katoris water

Method

Wash the mint and basil leaves thoroughly, then throw the leaves in 8 katoris of simmering water. When the water reduces to half its quantity, take it off the flame. Strain out the leaves and sip hot.

LEMON GRASS TEA 6 katoris (3 cups)

A really refreshing, fragrant infusion, to be enjoyed warm.

Ingredients

1 katori chopped lemon grass
2 cloves and cardamoms each, crushed (optional)
1 inch fresh ginger
8 katoris water

Method

Put all the ingredients in the 8 katoris of boiling water. Simmer on a low flame for about 5 minutes, or until the flavours get mixed in the water. Sip hot.

NUTRI BOWL RECIPES

Allowance = 2 katoris (1 cup)

MIXED VEGETABLE SOUP 8 katoris (4 cups)

Delicious mixed veggie soup, which you can vary by adding veggies in slightly different proportions, depending on what's available in your fridge.

Ingredients

1 medium size yellow pumpkin
1 medium size white pumpkin
1 medium carrot
3–4 florets cauliflower
1 bunch spinach leaves
1 onion
6 katoris water
salt to taste
choice of herbs

Method

Wash and cut the all vegetables. Boil the water in a vessel, and when it boils, add the vegetables. Cook the vegetables until soft but not mushy. Cool the vegetables and puree in a mixer/grinder. Add all the vegetable water to the pureed mixture.

Pour out the pureed liquid back into the cooking vessel. Season with dried oregano, basil, pepper and any herbs of your choice. Add fresh coriander if you wish. Serve hot.

MINT & CORIANDER LASSI 8 katoris (4 cups)

Beat the heat with a refresher that really quenches your thirst!

Ingredients

4 katoris low-fat curd
4 katoris water
¼ teaspoon ginger paste
1 teaspoon chopped mint leaves
1 teaspoon chopped coriander leaves

¼ teaspoon roasted, ground cumin
chaat masala (optional)
salt to taste

Method

Blend the curds and chaat masala, cumin powder, ginger and salt in a mixer till frothy. Add finely chopped mint and coriander to the lassi drink. Add ice cubes, or extra water, if required. Pour into a tall glass, and decorate with a sprig of mint. Enjoy cold.

MODIFIED GUJARATI KADHI 8 katoris (4 cups)

A twist to the traditional kadhi, that loses none of the flavour, but only the fat!

Ingredients

3 katoris sour low-fat curd
2 tablespoons yellow moong dal flour
5 katoris water
1 inch ginger, finely chopped
2–3 curry leaf stalks
¼ katori coriander leaves
2 green chillies, slit
salt to taste

For tempering

1 inch cinnamon
5 cloves
½ teaspoon mustard seeds
½ teaspoon fenugreek (methi) seeds
½ teaspoon cumin seeds
½ teaspoon asafoetida powder

Method

Combine the curds and moong dal powder, then whip to a creamy consistency. Add the water gradually, making sure there are no lumps. Then add the finely chopped ginger and salt to taste. Put this mixture to boil over a low flame. Stir to avoid lumps.

Slit the green chillies and chop the coriander, and keep them aside.

Dry roast the mustard seeds, cumin seeds, cinnamon, cloves, fenugreek seeds and curry leaves. Add slit green chillies and asafoetida. If it burns, you can add a few drops of water. Once the dry tadka is well roasted, drop it into the boiling kadhi.

Top the kadhi with freshly chopped green coriander, and serve hot with your recommended rice serving.

FRESH TOMATO SOUP 8 katoris (4 cups)

Cooked tomatoes are a wonder vegetable, with a very high lycopene content. However, tomatoes can be acidic, so fresh celery helps to counter the acidity.

Ingredients

10 fresh, ripe red tomatoes
1 medium onion
2–3 stalks celery
6 katoris water
salt & pepper to taste
fresh basil leaves (optional)

Method

Boil all the vegetables in a saucepan of water, till they become soft and pulpy. When the mixture cools, mash through a coarse sieve, until only the skin and seeds remain in the sieve.

Discard the skin and seeds, and put the pureed tomato soup back into the pan. Season with salt and pepper, garnish with fresh basil leaves. Simmer gently just before serving. Serve hot.

TOM YUM SOUP 8 katoris (4 cups)

A version of the typical tom yum soup that does not use oil, but tastes just as good.

Ingredients for the stock

1 katori roughly chopped cabbage
1 katori roughly chopped carrots
3–4 cauliflower florets
I chopped onion
6 katoris water

Ingredients for the soup

1 green chilli, cut length-wise
½ katori fresh mushrooms, sliced
1 katori carrot strips
1 katori chopped spring onions
2 teaspoons chopped celery
1 tablespoon finely chopped lemon grass stems
1 teaspoon lime juice
salt to taste

Method

Boil all the stock vegetables in 6 katoris of water. Once the vegetables are well-cooked, in about 20 minutes, discard the vegetables and save the stock for the soup.

Then add the chopped veggies to the stock, add in the green chillis, mushrooms, carrot strips, spring onions, celery, lemon grass and salt to taste. Simmer for 4–5 minutes. Stir in lime juice.

Serve hot with chillis and vinegar.

VEGETABLE JUICE 8 katoris (4 cups)

If you want more zing to your veggie juice, add radish, or a dash of Tabasco sauce.

Ingredients

1 medium size lauki (white gourd)
1 medium carrot
1 small bunch spinach leaves
1 tomato
1 stalk celery
2 teaspoons lime juice
4 katoris water
salt/rock salt to taste

Method

Wash and cut all the vegetables. Puree the vegetables in a food processor, then strain through a coarse sieve. This juice will make about 4 katoris. Add another 4 katoris of water to make 8 katoris. Add in the lime juice and salt. Consume immediately.

FIBRE FILLER RECIPES

Allowance = 2 katoris (1 cup)

I have compiled some interesting FIBRE FILLER recipes here. This can give you an idea of how much variety there is. You can use the veggies steamed or raw, or even go for a part-steamed, part-raw combination. Fruit can also be combined in novel ways, to give your palate something different every time. Pick fresh produce that is in season and locally available to get the maximum nutritional benefit from your FIBRE FILLER.

Did you know? Tomato is actually a fruit and not a vegetable. And yes, cauliflower is a real flower, and also a relative of the broccoli!

TOMATO AND LETTUCE MEDLEY 4 katoris (2 cups)

A great summer salad with a tangy freshness that tickles the palate.

Ingredients

8–10 large iceburg lettuce leaves, torn to bite size pieces
4 medium tomatoes cubed
1 teaspoon dried mango powder (amchur)
1 tablespoon chopped spring onions
1 teaspoon lemon juice (optional)
1 teaspoon cumin powder
rock salt to taste

Method

Toss up all the ingredients in a glass bowl. Chill for at least 5 minutes before serving.

CHATPATA KACHUMBAR 4 katoris (2 cups)

A heady combination of crunchy veggies, spiced just right!

Ingredients

1 katori sliced onions
2 katoris cucumber, sliced thin
1 katori sliced tomatoes
½ teaspoon roasted cumin powder (jeera)
¼ teaspoon chilli powder
1 teaspoon lemon juice
salt to taste

Method

Combine all ingredients in a large salad bowl. Serve immediately.

THAI PINEAPPLE CUCUMBER SALAD 4 katoris (2 cups)

This one has a Far Eastern flavour you will love.

Ingredients
1 katori fresh pineapple, diced
1 katori cucumber, diced
12–15 cherry tomatoes, halved
1 katori lettuce, shredded
2 tablespoons chopped coriander
2 tablespoons lemon juice
few sprigs Thai basil leaves, chopped
salt and freshly ground pepper to taste

Method
Combine all the salad ingredients in a large salad bowl. Toss lightly. Serve immediately.

CRUNCHY VEGETABLE SALAD 4 katoris (2 cups)

A colourful and flavourful salad to make your mouth water! The orange and lemon dressing packs in loads of vitamin C and you can combine any crunchy vegetables you find in your refrigerator.

Ingredients for the salad
1 katori red cabbage shredded
1 katori green cabbage shredded
1 katori thinly sliced carrots
½ katori white radish (mooli) thinly sliced
½ katori capsicum thinly sliced

Ingredients for the dressing
2 tablespoons orange juice
1 teaspoon lemon juice
¼ teaspoon prepared mustard
salt and pepper to taste

Method
Combine all salad ingredients in a glass bowl and refrigerate. Stir together all the dressing ingredients and store in a jar in the fridge. Just before serving, shake up the dressing in the bottle and pour over the salad. Toss well and serve.

READY RADISH 4 katoris (2 cups)

For radish lovers this is a real treat. The cumin-coriander sauce takes the 'bite' off the radish, yet enhances its naturally pungent flavour.

Ingredients

2 large radishes, (mooli) washed and scraped

Ingredients for the sauce

2 katoris fresh coriander, chopped
1 teaspoon cumin powder (jeera)
1 teaspoon onion seeds (kalonji)
2 tablespoons lime juice
rock salt to taste

Method

Make a paste of the sauce ingredients. (Please note the sauce, in paste form, will fill about ½ a katori.) Cut the radish into julienne strips. Mix the radish into the sauce and let it stand for 15 minutes.

Serve cold, or at room temperature.

FRUIT CHAAT 4 katoris (2 cups)

It's sweet, it's sour, it's spicy, it's simply delicious! Fruit lovers will rejoice at the medley of flavours that tease their palate.

Ingredients

1 guava, diced
1 sweet lime (mosambi) in segments
1 apple, diced
1 pear, diced
2 rings pineapple, diced
½ katori chopped coriander
1 green chilli, chopped fine (optional)
2 teaspoons lime juice
2 teaspoons chaat masala
2 teaspoons extract of tamarind
salt to taste

Method

Combine all the ingredients in a bowl and mix well. Serve immediately.

MAIN COURSE DINNER
VEGETABLE RECIPES

Allowance 1 katori (½ cup) = 1 serving

Cauliflower in onion chutney
Curried cucumber

Tandoori tinda
Grilled veggies
Stir-fried veggies Chinese style

CAULIFLOWER IN ONION CHUTNEY 4 servings 4 katoris (2 cups)

Not many know about the nutritional benefits of cauliflower—it is packed with vitamin C. This unusual recipe adds a sharp taste to the vegetable and gives you cauliflower with a new twist.

Ingredients

3 katoris grated cauliflower
1 green chilli without seeds, chopped fine
1 tablespoon fresh chopped coriander

Ingredients for the chutney

2 katoris chopped onion
2 katoris chopped tomato
2 cloves garlic
1 teaspoon cumin powder
¼ teaspoon pepper powder
rock salt to taste

Grind together the ingredients for the chutney into a fine paste. (Please note ground chutney will constitute 1 katori.) Combine this paste with the grated cauliflower and chopped green chillis. Mix well. Garnish with fresh coriander.

CUCUMBER/WHITE GOURD IN GREEN SAUCE 4 servings 4 katoris (2 cups)

A summery delight you will relish. The fresh, green look gives you a straight-out-of-the-garden feel—enjoy!

Ingredients

2 katoris diced cucumber/white gourd lightly steamed
1 ½ katoris raw mango, chopped fine (optional)

Ingredients for the sauce

1 katori fresh coriander
1 katori chopped mint
1 inch piece ginger
1 teaspoon cumin powder
1 green chilli chopped
rock salt to taste

Method

Grind the sauce ingredients to a paste. Mix the diced cucumber thoroughly with the sauce. Serve warm.

TANDOORI TINDA 4 servings 4 katoris (2 cups)

Many consider tinda dull and boring, but when you try this recipe, you will taste this humble vegetable in a new avatar.

Ingredients

- ½ kilo tinda (3 katoris)
- ½ teaspoon turmeric powder (haldi)
- ½ teaspoon jeera powder
- ½ teaspoon red chilli powder
- 1 teaspoon tandoori masala
- 1 teaspoon raw mango powder (amchoor)
- 1 katori cabbage shredded
- ½ teaspoon oil

Method

Wash and cut the tinda into small pieces. In ½ teaspoon of oil, add all the masala powders till they are well roasted. Add the tinda and shredded cabbage, fry to a light golden colour. Cook until vegetables are soft and till water from the vegetables dries up. Serve hot.

GRILLED VEGGIES 4 servings 4 katoris (2 cups)

A very versatile veggie option, where you can experiment with different veggie and herb combinations.

Ingredients

- 1 medium eggplant, cut lengthwise into quarters
- 1 medium zucchini or summer squash, cut lengthwise into quarters
- 3–4 portobello mushrooms
- ½ teaspoon olive oil
- mixed dried herbs—basil, oregano, thyme
- salt and freshly ground pepper

Method

Rub the prepared vegetables with olive oil, pepper, salt and herbs. Place in a single layer on the grill-rack over medium-high heat. Cook to desired state of doneness, turning as needed, until crisp-tender and flecked with brown.

(You may substitute portobello with other mushrooms, or add other veggies, like red onions, or bell peppers in different colours)

Ideas for leftover grilled veggies

1. Use chopped leftover grilled veggies as a nutritious and flavourful topping for couscous, pulao, brown rice, or other whole grains.
2. Mix grilled veggies with salsa and fill into a Mexican burrito.

STIR-FRIED VEGGIES CHINESE STYLE 4 servings 4 katoris (2 cups)

Savour all the delicious flavours of crunchy-cooked vegetables, with just the bare minimum of seasoning.

Ingredients

1 bunch bok choy
6 mushrooms, sliced
12 pieces baby corn
2 celery stalks, chopped diagonally
1 bunch green onions, chopped diagonally
1 inch piece fresh ginger, chopped fine
6 water chestnuts (optional)
1 teaspoon soy sauce
½ teaspoon black pepper
1 teaspoon oil

Method

Heat oil in a wok. (You can use a kadhai as a wok substitute.) Add the chopped ginger and stir for ½ a minute. Then add all the other vegetables, along with the soya sauce and pepper, and stir quickly on high heat, for 3 to 4 minutes. Take wok off the fire when the veggies are still crisp. Eat immediately.

RECIPES FOR PROTEIN-RICH OPTION

Allowance = 1 protein-rich serving for Plan Minimum & Medium
2 protein-rich servings for Plan Maximum

Herbed & grilled fish
Roast tandoori chicken
Moong sprout curry
Paneer bhurji

Tofu stir-fry
Yellow moong dal

HERBED & GRILLED FISH 4 servings

A delicious and simple way to eat fish, where fish-lovers can enjoy the subtle flavours of lime and herbs along with their favourite fish.

Ingredients

1 medium-sized pomfret
2 pods crushed garlic
juice of ½ lime
mixed dried herbs—basil, thyme, dill
salt & pepper to taste

Method

Rub the fish with lime juice, salt, crushed garlic and mixed herbs. Marinate for at least ½ an hour. Preheat oven to 250°C. Place the fish on a grilling tray, over a piece of tin foil.

Pop the tray into the hot oven. Using a flat spatula, gently turn over the fish after 10 minutes. Cook another 5 minutes, then put oven on browning mode for 3–4 minutes and brown the fish before serving.

Note: you can substitute pomfret with sole, cod, rawas or surmai.

ROASTED TANDOORI CHICKEN 4 servings

A succulent, spicy chicken preparation that needs no introduction. You will be amazed how, even without oil, the marinade tenderizes the meat to perfection. You can try this recipe as a fish version too, using any firm fish of your choice.

Ingredients

2 full chicken breasts, boneless, skinless

Ingredients for the marinade

½ teaspoon garlic paste
½ teaspoon ginger paste
2 teaspoons tandoori masala powder
½ teaspoon lime juice
salt & pepper to taste

Wash and clean the chicken breasts, then make diagonal slashes across with a sharp knife. Rub the marinade over the chicken breasts, allowing the marinade to seep in. Keep aside for at least 2 hours.

Method

Heat oven to 350°C. Place the chicken breasts on a foil tray, cover with tin foil and put into the oven. Cook for 20–25 minutes. Remove foil, allow to brown on both sides.

Cut the chicken breasts into 2 halves, 4 pieces in total, to make one serving each.

MOONG SPROUT CURRY 4 servings 4 katoris (2 cups)

While no lentils except moong are recommended on this diet, when a pulse or bean is sprouted, it becomes much lighter to digest. This is a delicious curry, in a spicy, chatpata masala gravy.

Ingredients

4 katoris sprouted moong
1 medium sized onion
½ teaspoon garlic-ginger paste
small pinch asafoetida (hing)
handful curry leaves
½ teaspoon mustard seeds
1 tablespoon tamarind extract
½ teaspoon red chilli powder
½ teaspoon jeera-dhania
¼ teaspoon turmeric (haldi)
½ teaspoon oil
salt to taste
½ katori fresh green coriander, chopped
1 green chilli (de-seeded), slit length-wise

Method

Heat the oil in a kadhai. Temper with hing, mustard seeds, garlic-ginger paste and curry leaves. Then add the onion. When onion is soft, add all the masala powders. Baste masala for a couple of minutes, then add the sprouted moong. Adjust the seasoning.

Add tamarind extract and simmer for 5 minutes, till the moong is cooked soft, but not over-cooked. Take off the fire, decorate with green chillis and coriander. Serve hot.

PANEER BHURJI 4 servings 4 katoris (2 cups)

You simply can't go wrong! A classic paneer bhurji, well-seasoned and well-browned—bhunaoed—is truly a delight. Delicious with rotis or, for a change, try it on wholewheat toast.

Ingredients

16 cubes low-fat paneer, of 1 inch x 1 inch each, crumbled (4 cubes per serving)
2 medium-sized onions, chopped fine
2 medium-sized tomatoes, chopped
1 teaspoon cumin seeds
¼ teaspoon turmeric (haldi)
½ teaspoon red chilli powder
1 teaspoon jeera-dhania powder
½ teaspoon garam masala
¼ cup chopped green coriander
1 teaspoon oil
salt to taste

Method

Heat oil in a kadhai. Add the cumin seeds. When cumin seeds go brown, add chopped onion. Cook onion till it is transparent, then add the chopped tomatoes. Once the tomatoes go pulpy, add all the masala powders. Stir this mixture till the masalas give off a great aroma. Then add the crumbled paneer. Add salt and mix well, adjust the seasoning if required. Cook for another 2–3 minutes.

Take the paneer dish off the fire, mix in the chopped green coriander, and serve hot.

TOFU STIR FRY 4 servings 4 katoris (2 cups)

The subtle, delicate tofu absorbs any flavour you add, so use the extras sparingly. Tofu dishes combine well with rice or noodles.

Ingredients

16 cubes of low-fat tofu, cut into 1 inch x 1 inch pieces (4 cubes per serving)
1 teaspoon soya sauce
¼ teaspoon red chilli powder
¼ teaspoon black pepper coarsely ground
½ teaspoon sesame oil (til oil)
1 bunch green onion, chopped fine
1 teaspoon roasted sesame seeds

Method

Heat the sesame oil in a flat pan. Add the tofu cubes and fry to a golden colour on all sides. Add the soya sauce, chilli powder and pepper. Lightly sauté for 1 minute, without breaking the tofu pieces.

Take the pan off the fire, transfer to flat serving dish. Garnish with chopped green onions and roasted sesame seeds. Serve hot.

YELLOW MOONG DAL 4 servings 4 katoris (2 cups)

Nothing like a katori of creamy-cooked, lightly tempered yellow moong dal to make your meal. Its hearty goodness brings to mind the simplicity of rustic fare—all you need is hot rotis, or rice, to do full justice!

Ingredients

2 katoris split yellow moong dal, soaked
3 katoris water
pinch turmeric
2 medium-sized onions, chopped fine
½ teaspoon whole cumin
½ teaspoon asafoetida
2 bay leaves (tej patta)
½ teaspoon garam masala
fresh chopped green coriander

Method

Boil the moong dal in 3 katoris of water, along with salt and turmeric. Roast the chopped onions in a kadhai, add the bay leaves, asafoetida and cumin seeds. Once the cumin seeds are well-roasted, add the cooked dal. Sprinkle with garam masala, adjust the seasoning.

Simmer dal mixture for 5 minutes. Serve hot, garnished with chopped coriander.

3-in-1 DINNER RECIPES

Allowance for Plan Minimum = ½ serving cereal + 1 serving fruits & veggies + 1 serving protein-rich food

Allowance for Plan Medium = 1 serving cereal + 1 serving fruits & veggies + 1 serving protein-rich foods

Allowance for Plan Maximum = 1 serving cereal + 1 serving fruits & veggies + 2 servings protein-rich foods

Grilled sandwich
Salad curd rice
Moong sprout bhel
Greek salad with garlic bread
Chicken kathi roll

GRILLED SANDWICH 4 servings—allowance for Plan Medium (please refer to your allowance if you are on Plan Minimum or Plan Maximum)

The bread gives you your cereal, the vegetable filling completes your veggie quota, and the paneer your high protein component. A very nutritious dinner, ready in no time at all.

Ingredients

4 large slices whole wheat bread
1 medium onion, chopped fine
2 medium tomatoes, chopped fine
1 capsicum, chopped fine
½ teaspoon jeera-dhania masala
¼ teaspoon ground pepper
16 pieces low-fat paneer cubes, 1 inch x 1 inch, crumbled
1 teaspoon butter
1 teaspoon oil
salt to taste

Method

Heat 1 teaspoon oil in a kadhai, cook onion and tomato to a pulpy consistency. Add the powder masalas and salt, blend well. Then add the crumbled paneer, stir. Adjust seasoning to taste.

Lightly butter the bread slices and place them buttered side down on a plate. Then, heap the paneer mixture evenly on 2 of the open slices. (Buttered side remains down.) Use the remaining 2 slices to cover the lower slices, like a sandwich, making sure the buttered side is on the outer side facing up.

This sandwich can be toasted in a sandwich toaster, or simply put onto a hot pan to brown. On a pan, toast the slices to a crisp golden brown on one side, then flip over, to brown on other side. (If you are using a pan, you may need to seal the inner edges by lining the inner side with a few drops of water before it goes onto the pan.) In a sandwich toaster, remove from toaster when golden brown.

Cut each sandwich into two triangles, giving you a total of four triangles. One triangle is one serving.

SALAD CURD RICE

4 servings—allowance for Plan Medium (please refer to your allowance if you are on Plan Minimum or Plan Maximum)

A delectable 3-in-1 option, with rice as the cereal component, the vegetables coming from the tomato-cucumber combination, and protein requirement from the yoghurt. This cooling dinner is perfect for a hot summer night!

Ingredients

4 katoris cooked rice
4 katoris low-fat curd
2 tomatoes, diced
1 cucumber, peeled and diced
2 slices pineapple, diced (optional)

Ingredients for the tempering

½ teaspoon mustard seeds
handful curry leaves
1 teaspoon urad dal
pinch asafoetida (hing)
1 teaspoon oil/ghee
salt to taste

Method

Mix rice and curds. Add the diced vegetables and salt, and blend in all the ingredients thoroughly. Keep aside.

In a small kadhai, heat the oil and add all the tempering ingredients. When this is crisp fried, add to the rice and curd mixture. Mix well and serve at room temperature. If you want to eat it cold, store in the refrigerator for about 1 hour.

MOONG SPROUT BHEL 4 servings—allowance for Plan Medium (please refer to your allowance if you are on Plan Minimum or Plan Maximum)

A 'fast food' 3-in-1 choice! Cereal comes from the puffed rice and vegetables from the fresh chopped tomato, onion and capsicum and green coriander chutney. Protein is complete with the moong sprouts—you can't believe low-fat bhel could be this delicious!

For the chutney
2 katoris green coriander
2 katoris mint leaves (pudina)
4 tablespoons lime juice
4 green chillis
2 teaspoons jeera (cumin)
salt to taste

For the bhel
4 katoris sprouted moong
2 cups salted water
8 katoris puffed rice (kurmura)
1 small onion, chopped fine
1 small cucumber, chopped fine
1 small capsicum, chopped fine
1 small tomato, chopped fine
2 green chillis, chopped fine
1 katori green coriander, chopped
rock salt or black salt to taste

First prepare the chutney. Puree all the ingredients to a fine paste. Keep aside.

Boil the moong sprouts in 2 cups of salted water. Drain out the water. (Do not throw out the water, as it makes a great Starter Sip for you.) Mix the sprouts with all the other bhel ingredients and top with green chutney. Eat immediately.

GREEK SALAD WITH GARLIC BREAD 4 servings—allowance for Plan Medium (please refer to your allowance if you are on Plan Minimum or Plan Maximum)

The cereal component comes from the delicious garlic bread croutons. Crunchy lettuce, onion and olives make up your vegetable

portion. The feta and cottage cheese completes the protein requirement, and the olive oil comes with its heart-friendly benefits, making this nutrition-packed 3-in-1 combo!

Ingredients

large bunch romaine lettuce leaves
16 cubes low-fat feta cheese, each 1 inch x 1 inch size
8 black olives, pitted
1 red onion, diced
2 ripe red tomatoes, diced
1 teaspoon balsamic vinegar
½ teaspoon coarsely crushed pepper
4–5 cloves garlic, chopped fine
2 teaspoons olive oil
4 large slices whole wheat bread (for the croutons)
salt to taste

Method

In a large glass bowl, tear the lettuce leaves and crumble the feta. Add diced olives and onion. Drizzle with balsamic vinegar, half the olive oil (1 teaspoon), add salt and pepper, mix all the ingredients well. Chill in refrigerator.

Mix the remaining olive oil, chopped garlic and salt in a small bowl. Spread this mixture onto the bread slices, on both sides. Cut the bread slices into 1 inch squares and toast on a hot pan, till they go crisp and golden brown. When these bread croutons cool, blend into the chilled salad and serve immediately.

CHICKEN KATHI ROLL 4 servings—allowance for Plan Medium (please refer to your allowance if you are on Plan Minimum or Plan Maximum)

This is like a low-cal version of the chicken Frankie, only far healthier. A non-vegetarian staple that travels well!

Ingredients

4 small rotis/phulkas

Ingredients for the filling

2 onions
4 teaspoons tomato paste
1 teaspoon ginger-garlic paste
1 teaspoon jeera dhania powder
1 teaspoon chilli powder
2 teaspoons oil

4 chicken breast pieces, 3 inch x 3 inch each
½ cup fresh green coriander chopped
1 katori shredded carrot/ cabbage
2 green chillis, chopped fine
1 teaspoon chaat masala
salt to taste

Heat oil in a pan. Add onion, cook until transparent. Add the powdered masalas and masala paste, tomato paste, and salt. Baste masala till it is brown. Cut the chicken into bite-sized pieces and mix into the masala. Cook the chicken until well-browned.

Take one roti at a time. Fill each one with the chicken mixture. Top with chopped green coriander leaves, shredded vegetables and chopped green chillis. Sprinkle some chaat masala. Roll up each stuffed roti and wrap it in tin foil. One wrap is one serving.

FREEBIES		
mustard seeds	**cloves**	**onion**
chat masala	**cardamom**	**curry leaves**
turmeric	**cinnamon**	**green coriander**
dill (saunf)	**pepper**	**ginger**
coriander (dhania) powder	**nutmeg**	**mint leaves**
asafoetida	**balsamic vinegar**	**tamarind**
cumin (jeera) powder	**bay leaf**	**garlic**
sambar masala	**elaichi**	**green chillis**

garam masala	oregano	lime juice
rasam powder	chilli flakes	tomato paste
chilli powder	basil	
kasuri methi	vanilla	

FREEBIE RECIPES

Mint coriander chutney
Tamarind chutney
Tomato salsa
Balsamic salad dressing
Ginger & lime pickle

MINT CORIANDER CHUTNEY 1 katori

2 katoris washed, chopped coriander leaves
2 katoris washed, chopped mint leaves
1 small onion
2 cloves garlic
6 green chilllis, chopped
1 teaspoon cumin powder (jeera)
1 teaspoon lime juice
salt to taste

Combine all ingredients in a blender and puree to a smooth paste. Serve immediately.

TAMARIND CHUTNEY 2 katoris

2 katoris tamarind pulp, extracted
2 dates, pitted and chopped fine
1 teaspoon cumin powder
1 teaspoon chilli powder
salt to taste

To prepare chutney, mix all the ingredients. This chutney stores well in the refrigerator for up to one week.

TOMATO SALSA 2 katoris

6 ripe tomatoes, peeled and chopped
1 small onion, chopped fine
1 bell pepper, chopped fine
2 green chillis/jalapeno chillis, chopped fine (optional)
2 tablespoons vinegar
1 teaspoon chilli powder
salt to taste

Combine all ingredients, mix well. Garnish with coriander. Serve chilled.

BALSAMIC SALAD DRESSING 1 katori

½ katori balsamic vinegar
½ katori diluted lime juice
1 teaspoon mixed dried herbs (basil, oregano, Italian herbs)
salt to taste

Combine all the ingredients in a glass bottle. Tightly close the bottle cover and shake up the ingredients till well blended. Chill the bottle. Before serving, shake it up once again.

GINGER AND LIME PICKLE 1 katori

¾ katori fresh ginger root, chopped in small pieces
¼ katori fresh lime juice
1 teaspoon whole green peppercorns (optional)
1 teaspoon whole black peppercorns
2 green chillis, slit lengthwise
salt to taste

Combine all the ingredients, mix well. Store in a pickle jar.

CHAPTER 9

COUNTDOWN BREAKFAST

Jump-start your day

A hearty breakfast contributes more to your health than you can imagine. Nothing like a filling, fibre-rich breakfast to get your day off to a great start! That's why breakfast is so important. A good breakfast keeps you active right through the morning and prevents the glucose 'low' that you would experience on an empty stomach. When your body is well-fuelled, not only are you more energized, you are also more mentally alert.

How skipping breakfast made me fat

I have always been up at the crack of dawn to get ready for my early morning yoga-pilates classes. Three times a week, I conduct classes beginning at 7.00 a.m. On other week days, I conduct group fitness classes at 10 a.m. So who had time for breakfast?

Apart from the time constraint, I also felt the need to stay light, not bloated and heavy from a big breakfast, as I went into my teaching classes. From my point of view, a filling breakfast just didn't make sense.

Or so I thought. My cup of morning tea was 'breakfast' and straight after that I dashed off for my first set of classes. Over time, despite my active schedule, I found myself gaining weight. I was often cranky and irritable. This was because I had skipped breakfast and my energy levels had dipped. To top it all, I was on a fairly intense exercise schedule with my students, which meant, after classes, I would end up feeling really really hungry.

Noon-time then became an all-you-can-eat affair, with me devouring anything and everything that came my way. I did not realize it at the time, but this was how my body was trying to compensate for being denied! Even now, after all these years, I recall with embarrassment my no-holds-barred cravings for cheese toast and chocolate milkshakes. Now I know why.

Unfortunately, many of us share the same problem. We find reasons to skip breakfast. Lack of time is a standard excuse. But skipping breakfast is flawed logic. At breakfast-time, your body has been without food for around 12 hours. You need to kick-start your metabolism for the new day. At this point, if you do not eat a proper breakfast, your body, instead of getting into top gear, is going to hit a morning slump. Like me, you will then find yourself listless and lethargic all through the morning.

What's worse, breakfast skippers feel the need to binge during the latter half of the day, to make up for lost time!

While I was working on my diet programmes, I came upon a study conducted by researchers at the University of California, Berkeley. This reveals that people who eat breakfast have significantly lower body mass index measurements than people who skip breakfast.

Today, my breakfast habits have changed completely. I prepare my own balanced breakfast, based on the 1, 2, 3 Formula, and make the time to eat it, and enjoy it. Now, I'm leaner, fitter and according to my students, much more cheerful in class!

CALORIE ALERT

Steer clear of sugary breakfast cereals, rich puri-bhaji or oily paratha options, buttery toast, doughnuts, jalebis. Spreads like syrups, jams and cream cheese are a diet no-no. Processed foods, such as white bread, are digested quickly and will leave you hungry and tired in a couple of hours.

WAKE UP TO WATER

Did you know that most people only drink about 3 to 4 glasses of water a day? How many glasses can you count for yourself? If your water consumption is anything below 8 glasses a day, you are under-hydrated.

About 65 per cent to 70 per cent of your body is made up of water, which is why you need a minimum 8 glasses of water for your body to function efficiently. Lack of water can cause severe problems such as dehydration, low blood pressure, constipation and poor metabolic function. Even mild dehydration can prevent the kidneys from effectively purifying the blood, which means toxins will keep building up in your system. Symptoms like nausea or drowsiness can accompany these conditions.

Remember: the best nutrient for weight loss is water. It has no fat, no carbohydrates, no calories, no sugar. It works as an appetite suppressant. Very often, when you think you are hungry, you are actually thirsty. So make the most of water; make it your diet ally.

FACT FILE

Excess salt can cause water retention and increase blood pressure. Restrict salt to 6 g, roughly about 1 teaspoon, per day. Substitute extra salt with herbs and spices such as oregano, basil, coriander and parsley, or use seasonings like lemon, garlic or pepper.

HOW DO YOU KNOW YOU ARE GETTING ENOUGH WATER?

The colour of your urine is a good indicator of your hydration levels. If you are drinking enough fluids, the urine will be almost clear in colour. The less water you drink, the darker your urine will become. (Please note that some medications may affect the colour of your urine.)

DURING THE COUNTDOWN, EVERY GLASS COUNTS

Water is so important thar you must start your day with a glass of water first thing in the morning. You can have your water warm with lemon, slightly chilled, or at room temperature. Gradually, learn to build up your water consumption to 2 glasses before breakfast.

Sip the warm lemon water slowly, giving your body about 30 minutes to digest this before breakfast. Lemon water is a great source of vitamin C and also stimulates the bowels.

Bonus points with early morning water

Shining hair
Glowing skin
Sparkling eyes

FACT FILE

Green tea works well as a water substitute, because it has no caffeine. It can be enjoyed all through the day to aid digestion, and is especially effective after a meal. Green tea is also rich in flavonoids—plant pigments that protect against infection.

To give you the maximum benefit from the 1, 2, 3 Formula, your COUNTDOWN breakfast comes served up with high-energy carbs, packed with vitamins and minerals, loaded with body building proteins . . . and some fabulous breakfast ideas!

The best part is that the breakfast choices are all yours. Whether you are in the mood for a Gujarati type naashta, a South Indian style tiffin, or a classic English breakfast, your COUNTDOWN breakfast wakes up your taste buds like never before.

Good morning, and have a happy breakfast!

1, 2, 3 Formula Breakfast

1. CEREAL SERVING for your carbohydrate energy boost. Try to pick fibre-rich cereal options for a healthier breakfast.

FIBRE FOR BREAKFAST

Certain fibre-rich cereals such as oats, whole-grain bread, dalia or bran flakes make great low-cal breakfast options. The bulk these cereals provide supports your weight-loss efforts, because each of these high-fibre options fills you up and keeps you full for a longer period of time.

Fibre also helps to stimulate lazy bowels. Do remember: fibre requires ample water to function optimally, so make sure you increase your fluids to help fibre to move more smoothly through the intestines.

2. FRUIT or VEGETABLE for your vitamin and mineral requirements. Vary the colour of your fruits and vegetables, as different colours give you different nutrients.

TO PEEL OR NOT TO PEEL

Eating the skin of certain vegetables and fruits ensures a higher fibre intake. For example, in an apple, the peel contains 75 per cent of the dietary fibre. If you decide to eat the peel, make sure the fruits and vegetables are properly washed. Another important point: fruit is best consumed whole, not as fruit juice. Fruit juice is not only higher in calories, it also deprives you of valuable fibre.

3. MILK or NUTS & SEEDS or EGGS are some protein-rich options. Animal sources such as milk, milk products, meats and eggs are complete sources of proteins, containing all the essential amino acids. Vegetarian proteins are incomplete and need to be combined with other foods to be complete. Protein-rich vegetarian foods include pulses, soya products, nuts and seeds.

NOTE: Restrict whole eggs to no more than 2 eggs per week, as egg yolks are high in cholesterol and calories. Egg whites, however, can be consumed daily if desired.

½ TEASPOON FAT

When you prepare your basic COUNTDOWN breakfast, you are allowed a ½ teaspoon of any fat of your choice. It could be butter on your toast or ghee in your upma—the choice is yours, but do not exceed your allowance!

BONUS BEVERAGE

You also get to have the hot or cold beverage that you would normally consume. If you are a tea or coffee drinker, you can have your morning cup that cheers, with skimmed milk and one teaspoon of sugar.

BREAKFAST FOR THE MORNING EXERCISER

If you exercise first thing in the morning, you may not want a big pre-exercise breakfast, as too much food can make you sluggish. But if a cup of coffee or tea won't suffice, feel free to have your cereal allowance, or your fruit or veggie option, along with your morning tea. You can then enjoy the rest of your COUNTDOWN breakfast after exercise.

BREAKFAST ON-THE-GO

Be creative about breakfast on-the-go and always think 1, 2, 3. For instance, a refreshing fruit and milk smoothie combines 2 and 3 components of the Formula. So what about 1, the cereal component? Carry any cereal of your choice, from crackers to roasted khakras, in a pouch. Top it up with coffee at the office.

Even something as simple as a vegetable sandwich works. Combine low-fat cottage cheese (paneer) with low-cal veggies in a sandwich, for a perfect 1, 2, 3 breakfast.

1. Toasted whole wheat bread slice/slices as per your allowance.
2. Sliced cucumber, mint chutney, tomato.
3. Low-fat cottage cheese (paneer) made from skimmed milk.

Sprinkle chilli flakes, pepper, or add mustard for extra taste, and make up a zesty sandwich. And hey, a 1, 2, 3 breakfast is ready to go, when you are!

BREAKFAST CHECK-IN

Choose your breakfast based on how much weight you need to lose. Please refer to my Plan Minimum, Plan Medium and Plan Maximum to slot yourself correctly.

Check your Daily Food Guide in Annexure B to understand 'What makes one serving?' This determines the serving size of cereal, fruit and veggie and protein-rich foods allowed for your particular Plan.

A quick reference guide is provided on the following page. For clarifications and more options, please refer to Annexure B.

PLAN MINIMUM breakfast

for women to lose up to 4 kilos

1 CEREAL **1 serving**

1 roti/1 large slice bread (made of any cereal)
or
1 katori ready-to-eat cereal/cooked cereal of your choice (cornflakes/wheatflakes/poha/upma)

+

2 FRUIT & VEGETABLE **1 serving**

1 katori of your choice (restrict potato, jackfruit, yam, banana, mango)

+

3 PROTEIN-RICH FOOD **1 serving**

1 katori moong sprouts
or
4 cubes low-fat paneer/low-fat feta cheese/tofu/1 katori low-fat curd
or
1 moong dal dosa/3 pieces dhokla/1 dosa/1 panki/1 chilla (made from 1 tablespoon moong flour)

or

1 medium-sized piece white meat (chicken breast/turkey breast/ fish)

or

2 egg whites/½ egg boiled

Bonus allowance 1 cup tea/coffee

PLAN MEDIUM breakfast

for men to lose up to 4 kilos and for women to lose 5–10 kilos

1 CEREAL 2 servings

2 rotis/2 large slices bread (made of any cereal)

or

2 katoris ready-to-eat cereal/cooked cereal of your choice (cornflakes/wheatflakes/poha/upma)

+

2 FRUIT & VEGETABLE 1 serving

1 katori of your choice (restrict potato, jackfruit, yam, banana, mango)

+

3 PROTEIN-RICH FOOD 1 serving

1 katori moong sprouts

or

4 cubes low-fat paneer/low-fat feta cheese/tofu/1 katori low-fat curd

or

1 moong dal dosa/3 pieces dhokla/1 dosa/1 panki/1 chilla (made from 1 tablespoon moong flour)

or

1 medium-sized piece white meat (chicken breast/turkey breast/ fish)

or
2 egg whites/½ egg boiled

Bonus allowance 1 cup tea/coffee

PLAN MAXIMUM breakfast
for men to lose more than 5 kilos; for women to lose more than 11 kilos

1 CEREAL 2 servings

2 rotis/2 large slices bread (made of any cereal)
or
2 katoris ready-to-eat cereal/cooked cereal of your choice (cornflakes/wheatflakes/poha/upma)

+

2 FRUIT & VEGETABLE 1 serving

1 katori of your choice (restrict potato, jackfruit, yam, banana, mango)

+

3 PROTEIN-RICH FOOD 1 serving

1 katori moong sprouts
or
4 cubes low-fat paneer/low-fat feta cheese/tofu/1 katori low-fat curd
or
1 moong dal dosa/3 pieces dhokla/dosa/panki/chilla (made from 1 tablespoon moong flour)
or
1 medium-sized piece white meat (chicken breast/turkey breast/fish)

or
2 egg whites/½ egg boiled

Bonus allowance 1 cup tea/coffee

Bonus allowance if drinking tea or coffee

tea/coffee with ½ serving low-fat milk + 1 teaspoon sugar
or
herbal tea
or
coconut water

SUGAR SUBSTITUTES

Many dieters opt for artificial sweeteners in their tea and coffee. The jury is still out on this one, with no conclusive proof that all sweeteners are harmful. In fact, some studies indicate that sugar substitutes may help in weight loss. I recommend minimal use of sugar and sugar substitutes, because controlling your cravings for sugar is the only long-term solution that works!

BREAKFAST RECIPES

1 katori = ½ cup = 100 grams
2 katoris = 1 cup = 200 grams

The 1, 2, 3 Breakfast suggestions here cater to serving allowances for Plan Medium and Plan Maximum. For breakfast, both

categories are the same. If you are following Plan Minimum, reduce the cereal serving by half. The remaining menu should be retained as it is.

1, 2, 3 BREAKFAST COMBO SUGGESTIONS

2 katoris (1 cup) dalia upma with vegetables + 2 katoris (1 cup) yoghurt
or
2 katoris (1 cup) oatmeal porridge with skimmed milk + 1 katori (½ cup) mixed fruit cup
or
2 whole wheat toasts + 1 vegetable omelette
or
2 katoris (1 cup) veggie poha + 2 katoris (1 cup) cold mocha coffee
or
1 moong dal dosa with tomato chutney + 1 vegetable cutlet sandwich

DALIA UPMA WITH VEGETABLES 4 servings 12 katoris (6 cups)

Dalia is a delicious and filling breakfast food, with multi-hued veggies to brighten up your morning! Please bear in mind the vegetable serving is one katori, so you will eat three katoris (1 ½ cups) of upma.

Ingredients

6 katoris broken wheat dalia (soaked 8 katoris)
1 medium onion, chopped
2 carrots, diced
1 small capsicum, diced
1 katori (½ cup) corn kernels
½ inch piece grated ginger
3 slit green chillis
pinch asafoetida (hing)
pinch turmeric powder
½ teaspoon mustard seeds
handful curry leaves
2 teaspoons oil
4 katoris (2 cups) water
chopped coriander for garnish
2 tablespoons lime juice
salt to taste

Method

Roast dalia in a pan on low flame until light brown in colour. Remove from pan, keep aside. Heat the oil in a kadhai, add mustard seeds, asafoetida and curry leaves. When mustard seeds splutter, add grated ginger and slit green chillis.

Add chopped onion, stir. Then add other diced vegetables. Stir for about 5 minutes and add dalia. Season with salt and turmeric. Add 2 cups water and put in pressure cooker till dalia is soft and crumbly.

Blend in the lime juice and top with chopped coriander leaves. Serve hot.

MOCHA COLD COFFEE 4 servings 8 katoris (4 cups)

If you love the chocolate and coffee combo, this one's for you!

Ingredients

8 katoris low-fat milk, chilled
4 teaspoons sugar (this comes from your breakfast sugar allowance)
4 tablespoons instant coffee
4 tablespoons cocoa powder
1 teaspoon vanilla essence
a pinch cinnamon powder (for garnish)

Method

Whip up all the ingredients (except cinnamon powder) in a blender, until frothy. Pour into a tall glass, sprinkle with cinnamon powder. Serve chilled.

MOONG SPROUT CHAAT 4 servings 8 katoris (4 cups)

Crunchy, tangy breakfast option, guaranteed to wake you up and get you through a busy morning. Your protein comes from the katori of moong and the veggie requirement from the chopped mixed vegetables, adding up to two katoris per serving.

Ingredients

4 katoris sprouted moong, with skin (lightly steamed)
3 tomatoes, chopped
2 carrots, diced
2 capsicums, diced
1 large bunch green onions, chopped
½ teaspoon lime juice
1 teaspoon chaat masala
½ katori green coriander, chopped

Method

Steam the moong sprouts for 3–4 minutes, to retain the crunch. Cool the sprouts. Add all the other ingredients, mix well. Serve cold, or at room temperature.

NOTE: I have not added any extra salt, as chaat masala already contains salt. However, if you feel the dish is low on salt, add a small pinch.

MOONG DAL DOSA 4 servings, allowance at 1 dosa per serving

An extremely nutritious protein-rich dosa, originally from Andhra Pradesh. It goes very well with tomato chutney, and is a great breakfast option.

Ingredients

4 katoris green moong dal, soaked
1 large onion, chopped fine
2 finely grated carrots
2 inch piece ginger, grated
4–6 green chillies
1 large bunch green coriander leaves, chopped
2 teaspoons cumin seeds (jeera)
2 teaspoons oil
salt to taste

Method

Soak moong dal overnight. Grind together with ginger, chillies, coriander leaves and salt. Add finely chopped onion, carrot, and jeera to the dosa batter.

Heat a few drops of oil in a non-stick pan. Pour out batter, to make a medium-thick dosa. When one side is golden brown, flip over to brown other side. Serve hot with tomato chutney or garlic chutney.

POHA WITH PEAS AND CORN 4 servings 12 katoris (6 cups)

Traditional fare that makes a very satisfying breakfast. Remember, frozen peas are more tender and will cook faster than fresh peas.

Ingredients

6 katoris poha (8 katoris soaked)
1 ½ katori peas (boiled)
1 ½ katori corn (boiled)
2 large onions, chopped
½ teaspoon oil
¼ teaspoon mustard seeds
pinch asafoetida (hing)
handful curry leaves
3 slit green chillis
2 pods garlic, crushed (optional)
a pinch turmeric
2 teaspoons lime juice
large bunch green coriander chopped (for garnish)
4 katoris (2 cups) water
salt to taste

Method

Gently wash the poha in running water, then soak for 2–4 minutes. Lightly squeeze out the water, set aside. Heat oil in a kadhai, add mustard seeds, asafoetida, curry leaves, green chillis and garlic pods. Then add the onions and peas and corn, stir, and cook until onion is transparent.

Add the soaked poha, salt and turmeric. Mix all ingredients well, then add ¼ katori water, only if required. When water dries up, sprinkle lime juice, top with chopped green coriander. Serve hot.

VEGETABLE OMELETTE 4 servings

You can do a 'scrambled' version, by simply stirring up the egg-veggie mixture in the pan, like a bhurji. When it is ready, heap it on whole-wheat toast.

Ingredients

8 egg whites/2 full eggs
1 teaspoon milk
2 onions, finely chopped
3 tomatoes, finely chopped
1 red bell pepper, diced
1 yellow bell pepper, diced
1 large bunch coriander leaves, chopped

½ green chilli, finely chopped
3 olives, chopped (optional)
¼ teaspoon jeera dhania powder
¼ teaspoon red chilli powder
½ teaspoon olive oil/ghee
salt to taste

Method

Whip up eggs, milk and salt. Add all vegetables and continue beating until light and frothy. Then heat the oil, preferably use a non-stick pan. When oil is hot, pour in the egg-vegetable mixture. Cover the pan, and let the omelette cook, about 2–3 minutes. If you require it brown on both sides, flip over. Sprinkle with fresh pepper if desired. Serve hot.

VEGGIE CUTLET SANDWICH 4 servings with 2 slices per serving

Versatile vegetable cutlets are actually a non-messy and easy-to-make breakfast dish. You could keep the cutlet mixture ready in the fridge the night before, so all you do is shape and shallow fry the cutlets in the morning.

Ingredients

8 slices multigrain bread

Ingredients for the cutlet

3 katoris mixed veggies—carrots, french beans, cauliflower, celery
1 katori mashed potato
1 teaspoon cumin and coriander powder
1 teaspoon chilli powder
2 teaspoons lime juice
a pinch of turmeric
2 green chillis, finely chopped
1 teaspoon oil
salt to taste

Method

Lightly steam vegetables, until cooked but slightly crunchy. Mix into the mashed potatoes, add all the masalas and salt. Cook this mixture on a slow fire for about 5 minutes, until masalas are cooked and the water evaporates completely, to form a dough-like consistency. Shape the mixture into four cutlets.

Heat oil in a non-stick pan, shallow fry the cutlets till golden brown on both sides. Place each cutlet between 2 slices of bread, into a sandwich. One sandwich makes one serving. Serve with mint chutney.

BREAKFAST ON-THE-GO

If you need to get to your workplace and have to eat on the way, opt for something portable. Whatever you go with, remember, you must stay with the 1, 2, 3 Formula.

VEGETABLE & PANEER SANDWICH 4 servings, with 2 slices to make a sandwich

Ingredients

4 tomatoes, sliced in rounds
2 cucumber, sliced in rounds
6–8 lettuce leaves, washed and dried
16 cubes low-fat paneer, each 1 inch x 1 inch in size (4 cubes one serving)
8 slices whole-wheat bread
2 teaspoons butter
pepper and salt to taste

Method

Butter the bread slices. Place the tomato and cucumber slices on each one, season with salt and pepper. Crumble the paneer over the vegetables. Make up the sandwich, by placed one slice over the other.

NOTE: If you are with PLAN MINIMUM, you will use only one slice bread, either you can make it an open sandwich, or cut the slice into 2 triangles and make a half sandwich.

CHICKEN & VEGGIE WRAP 4 servings

Ingredients

8 rotis—for the wraps

Ingredients for the filling

4 pieces boiled or roasted chicken, each 3 inch x 3 inch in size
3–4 stalks celery, chopped
2 small onions/green onions, chopped
¼ cup coriander, chopped
4–5 olives, chopped
½ teaspoon pepper
1 teaspoon prepared mustard dressing

Method

Combine all the filling ingredients to make a spicy chicken mixture. Lay out the 8 rotis and place the chicken filling on the rotis, dividing equally. Roll up each roti, folding in the top and bottom edges to seal in the filling. Wrap in tin foil. Two rotis make one serving.

NOTE: Chicken can be substituted with roast turkey or water-packed tuna.

CHAPTER 10

COUNTDOWN IN-BETWEENS

Fill in the gaps

Your COUNTDOWN breakfast, lunch and dinner are all small meals and, chances are, you are going to feel quite hungry between these meals. So what do you do? Smart snacking is the way to go. Eating at frequent intervals stabilizes your blood sugar levels and keeps your metabolism fired up through the day.

Like most dieters, you might feel snacking during a diet seems bizarre. But before you see visions of yourself raiding the refrigerator, or feasting on samosas, burgers and chocolate cakes, let me quickly clarify! Your snacking, as with the rest of your COUNTDOWN, is controlled. It's called disciplined munching.

In-Betweens are also based on the 1, 2, 3 Formula. The only difference is, because In-Betweens are bite-size meals, you cannot have all the 3 food groups at one time. You therefore space out your 1, 2, 3 choices—cereals, fruits and vegetables and protein-rich foods—over 3 separate snacking sessions through the day.

So, for example, if you have a protein-rich option for your morning In-Between, then you go for a fruit or veggie option in the afternoon, and have a cereal option for early evening. On any given day, you can juggle around the 3 In-Betweens as you wish.

In-Betweens may not seem that important, but let me warn you, do not make the mistake of neglecting them! One of my clients, Amit Rele, stayed on track for breakfast, lunch and dinner, but In-Betweens were a huge challenge. He was so caught up with meetings, briefings, or looking into the next office crisis, In-Betweens were simply not on his list of priorities.

You could probably guess what happened next. Amit started ordering pakoras from the office canteen and grabbing burgers on the run. Before he realized it, Amit's diet was spinning out of control.

Like Amit, you and I lead busy lives. It's hard enough working to maintain our 3 main meals, let alone worry about In-Betweens! I couldn't agree more. But all I ask here is just a little bit of planning. It's not a big deal. Once you plan and prepare, you will find that your In-Betweens automatically fall into place.

HOW TO FILL THE LOGISTICS GAP

Zoom away with zip lock In-Betweens

Over time, I have learnt to use In-Betweens as an effective diet tool. Initially, I must confess the logistics gaps were huge. I would forget to pack my snack. Or, if I packed it, I would forget to eat it. Now, I make it a point to stock up on zip lock bags of all sizes, at all times. Zip locks are a great way to go. Slip them into purses and briefcases for instant access to any snack—fruit, sandwiches, wraps, sprouts—take your pick!

Alarm Timers

Another handy device is alarms. In the initial stages of your COUNTDOWN, alarms work as great In-Betweens reminders.

Simply set the timings on your cell phone, and every time your alarm goes off, you know you are due for your next In-Between.

FACT FILE

The longer your gap between meals, the hungrier you get, which means the more you are likely to overeat.

TIME IT RIGHT

As I mentioned earlier, In-Betweens are all about timing. Ideally, you should be eating something every two and a half hours. This is the recommended gap between meals. For example, if you have an early breakfast, say by 7.30 a.m., your **Mid Morning In-Between** could be around 10 a.m. This could be followed by lunch around 12.30 p.m.

But if you eat breakfast later, around 9.00 am, then your **Mid Morning In-Between** can wait till around 11.30 a.m. Naturally, in the real world, it is not possible to function exactly by the clock! As far as possible, try to get your schedule in place, so your In-Betweens fall into a set routine.

The **Afternoon In-Between** is your next snack, followed by an **Evening In-Between**. Try to adjust your In-Betweens in such a way that you allow a gap of two and a half hours, but no more than three hours every time you eat.

THE CASE OF THE MISGUIDED SNACKER

One of my newer clients, Nandita Mehta, a strict vegetarian, came to me when her earlier diet had backfired. She was seeing a dietician

KEEP YOUR WATER SUPPLY SWITCHED ON

Your body loses water all through the day and needs to be continuously re-hydrated. The minimum requirement of 8 glasses of water must be consumed at regular intervals. Try to finish your quota of 4 glasses, roughly 1 litre, by lunch time, and have the balance 4 glasses during the course of the day.

who had advised restricted consumption of dairy products as part of her weight loss plan. Nandita was encouraged to eat a low-calorie snack every two to three hours, to rev up her metabolism. She stocked up on packets of roasted farsans and baked namkeens from the health store and enjoyed her snacks at regular intervals through the day.

Three months into her diet, Nandita found she was losing hair and had become pale and listless. She felt completely drained out by the end of the day. Her physician evaluated her diet which was low in protein and vitamin B12. The restricted diet, with its limited nutrition, had taken its toll.

Nobody told Nandita that, unless she got her nutrients from different sources, losing weight could come with huge health risks. When her health began to suffer, Nandita realized the importance of a healthy, balanced diet plan.

To ease her back into a diet plan, I advised her to keep munching every two to three hours, but to munch sensibly. So Nandita switched to kurmura or roasted khakras mid-morning, 1 cup curd in the afternoon and a fruit in the evening. She enjoyed green tea or coconut water as her choice of beverage. In addition, she also included a portion of protein-rich food for breakfast, lunch and dinner. This new diet plan provided her with all-round nutrition. And the bonus? It kept her palate interested too!

I recently saw Nandita again. Her hair had re-gained its vitality and her skin was glowing. She had dropped a few kilos and was looking trim and fit. Much to my delight, she informed me that she had so much surplus energy, she had enrolled for salsa classes with her husband—living la vida loca!

IN-BETWEENS ARE THE SAME FOR
PLANS MINIMUM, MEDIUM & MAXIMUM

Beverage + Bite = Balanced In-Betweens

The beverage works as comfort food, filling you up with every sip and the bite is a small snack that comes loaded with nutrients. The combination keeps your hunger pangs under control until your next meal.

Mid Morning In-Between	**Beverage** 1 cup **+ Bite** 1 serving
Afternoon In-Between	**Beverage** 1 cup **+ Bite** 1 serving
Evening In-Between	**Beverage** 1 cup **+ Bite** 1 serving

List of Beverages for all 3 COUNTDOWN Diet Groups

CHOOSE YOUR BEVERAGE 2 katoris (1 cup)

skimmed milk
or
buttermilk

or

soup/rasam

or

vegetable juice

or

herbal tea or decaf tea or coffee

or

coconut water

or

coffee with ½ serving milk + 1 teaspoon sugar

or

plain tea/masala tea/cardamom tea/ginger tea with ½ serving milk + 1 teaspoon sugar

Note: Limit your tea/coffee to 2 cups a day, as it contains caffeine. This includes your morning allowance of tea/coffee with breakfast.

CHOOSE YOUR BITE

In the course of the day, you are allowed 3 Bites for your In-Betweens. Each time, you are required to exercise any ONE option from the 1,2,3 food groups. Your Bites should consist of one serving of cereal, or one serving of fruit or vegetable, or one serving of any protein-rich food. **There is no hard and fast rule about which Bite you choose for a particular In-Between.**

CEREAL BITE

2 katoris light savoury such as puffed rice

or

2 small roasted khakras

or

1 large slice bread

Looking for zip lock options? Carry along 2 non-creamy biscuits or 2 roasted khakras.

Dry cereal is great to munch on the go . . . zip lock it and zip away!

FRUIT & VEGETABLE BITE

1 katori mixed fruit/vegetable
or
1 fruit
or
3 dried fruits such as apricots, prunes or figs

In the mood for something zingy? Squeeze lime juice over your fruit and veggies, or sprinkle chaat masala and chilli powder to pep up your taste-buds!

PROTEIN-RICH FOOD BITE

5 nuts
or
1 katori curd
or
4 cubes low-fat paneer/low-fat feta cheese/tofu
or
1 katori moong dal/3 pieces dhokla/1 dosa/1 panki/1 chilla
or
1 medium-sized piece white meat—chicken breast/turkey breast/fish
or
2 egg whites

Craving something creamy? Just whip up your yoghurt portion, add a dash of vanilla essence or powdered elaichi for extra flavour.

IMPORTANT

FATS & SUGAR ALLOWANCE

For any one of the In-Between options, ½ a teaspoon of fat is allowed.

This may be in the form of butter, cooking oil, ghee or cream.

Your sugar allowance for the day is 2 teaspoons. Make it a point to keep a mental note of your daily consumption.

FREEBIES to enhance flavour	
Mint-coriander chutney	Oregano
Mustard	Chilli Flakes
Lime Juice	Basil Leaves
Vanilla	Ginger
Tamarind Chutney	Elaichi
Green Chillis	Cumin powder (jeera)
Chaat Masala	Garam Masala
Onion/Garlic	Tomato/Cucumber

Please note In-Betweens are the same for PLAN MINIMUM, PLAN MEDIUM & PLAN MAXIMUM dieters. Remember to rotate the 3 food groups through the day. Once during the day, you are allowed to add ½ a teaspoon of fat to any one of your In-Betweens.

Check your Daily Food Guide in Annexure B to understand 'What makes one serving?' This determines the serving size of cereal, fruit and veggie and protein-rich foods allowed for your particular Plan.

For more clarifications and options, please refer to Annexure B.

IN-BETWEENS RECIPES

1 katori = ½ cup = 100 grams
2 katoris = 1 cup = 200 grams

I have suggested a few In-Betweens options here.

CEREAL OPTIONS
allowance = 1 serving

Rava idli
Masala puffed rice (kurmura)
Whole wheat biscuits—2
Popcorn
Bajra dhokla
1 slice whole-grain bread/khakra/thepla with mint chutney

RAVA IDLI 4 servings

Ingredients

2 katoris wheat sooji/rava
1 ½–2 katoris water
½ teaspoon grated ginger
2 finely chopped green chilies
½ teaspoon soda bicarb
¼ cup grated carrot (optional)
2–3 sprigs coriander leaves, chopped fine
few drops lime juice
salt to taste

Method

Roast the rava lightly. Then add in all the ingredients and mix into a batter with water. Adjust the water to ensure a semi-liquid consistency, not too thin, not too thick, making sure there are no lumps. Keep aside for around 30 minutes.

Heat a pot of boiling water, then, in a greased idli stand, pour out the batter into four compartments, dividing equally, and place stand in the pot of boiling water. (You can also use a pressure cooker.)

Steam for around 15–20 minutes. When the idlis cool, spoon out each idli carefully. Serve with coriander chutney.

Option: For takeaway, pack idlis in zip lock pouch.

Bajra-raagi dhokla 4 servings

Ingredients

2 katoris bajra-raagi atta
1 teaspoon garlic paste
½ teaspoon green chilli paste
¼ teaspoon asafoetida
1 teaspoon soda bicarb
2 katoris water
small bunch coriander leaves, chopped
salt to taste

Method

Sift bajra-raagi atta in a bowl. Add soda bicarb, water, salt, asafoetida and water in it. Mix all these ingredients to make a thick batter. Keep this mixture aside for about 4 hours. Then add garlic and green chilli paste to the batter, mix well.

Next, boil some water in a pan. Meanwhile, lightly grease a shallow thali with oil, then pour the batter on it. Place the thali over the pan of boiling water and cover, letting the batter steam-cook in the thali.

After 10–15 minutes, insert a knife to check if dhoklas are cooked. Once the dhoklas are done, remove thali from heat and cool. Sprinkle the chopped coriander leaves on the top.

Bajra and raagi are power-packed grains, with high levels of iron and calcium. A mixed cereal diet is much better than a single cereal one, because different grains offer different nutritional benefits.

FRUIT & VEGGIE OPTIONS

allowance = 1 serving

Steamed veggies
Sliced cucumber & tomato slices with lemon
Stewed apple & pear
Corn-on-the-cob
Guava chaat

STEAMED VEGGIES 4 servings

Ingredients

2 carrots, cut in thick strips
handful French beans
4–6 florets cauliflower
4–6 florets broccoli
8 baby corn kernels

Method

Wash and cut vegetables into large pieces. Place in heated pan, with a little salt and pepper added. Cover the pan and let the veggies steam in their own juices. Add a few drops of water if the veggies are sticking at the bottom.

When vegetables are crunchy cooked, remove from fire and cool. Sprinkle chaat masala or chilli flakes on the veggies if desired.

For takeaway: Carry in zip lock bag or plastic container.

> Steaming vegetables preserves their flavours and nutrients, while boiled veggies lose most of their nutrition in the water, which gets thrown away.

GUAVA CHAAT 4 servings

Ingredients

4 medium-sized guavas
½ teaspoon chilli powder
1 teaspoon chaat masala
½ teaspoon lime juice

Method

Scoop out the seeds portion from the centre of the guava. Dice the guavas and sprinkle with chaat masala, chilli powder and lime juice.

PROTEIN-RICH OPTIONS

allowance = 1 serving

Chicken shake 'n' bake
Moong sprout medley
Paneer sautéed

CHICKEN SHAKE 'N' BAKE 4 servings

Ingredients

2 medium-sized chicken breasts, boneless, skinless
1 teaspoon soya sauce
1 teaspoon prepared mustard
2 teaspoons teriyaki sauce
2 teaspoons worcestershire sauce (optional)
salt to taste

Method

Cut the two chicken breasts into four pieces and pound each one to an even flatness.

Place the chicken pieces into a large zip lock pouch, add all the sauces into the pouch, and seal it up properly. Shake the bag, allowing all the sauces to blend together. Keep the pouch in the fridge for half an hour.

Heat your oven to 350°C. Get the bag out of the fridge and once again, shake vigorously. Then place the chicken pieces in a foil tray and bake for about ½ an hour, or until the chicken is thoroughly cooked. You can flip the pieces over once, for even browning.

MOONG SPROUT MEDLEY 4 servings

Ingredients

4 katoris sprouted moong steamed
2 tomatoes, chopped
1 large bunch green onion, chopped
2 teaspoons lime juice
a pinch chaat masala (optional)
1 green chilli, chopped fine
Salt to taste

Method

Toss all the ingredients together, mix well. Consume immediately.

PANEER SAUTEED 4 servings

Ingredients

16 cubes low-fat paneer, 1 inch x inch each (4 cubes make one In-Between Bite)
2 teaspoons green garlic, chopped fine (optional)
1 teaspoon oil
chilli flakes (optional)
½ teaspoon coarse-ground pepper
salt to taste

Method

Heat the oil and sauté the garlic in a non-stick pan. Add the paneer cubes and masalas. Saute for a couple of minutes. Enjoy hot.

WHEY PROTEIN

The liquid that separates from paneer solids is called whey. This milk by-product is rich in lactic acid as well as valuable proteins. When you make paneer, do not discard the whey. Instead, use it in soups, or mix it into chapati dough for added nutrition.

CHAPTER 11

COUNTDOWN LUNCH

A light meal goes a long way

It's lunchtime folks. Lunch, as we know it, comes in all shapes and sizes. Thali lunch, buffet lunch, dabba lunch, sandwich lunch, on-the-go lunch, weekend lunch, brunch, the list goes on. So what does your lunch look like?

Lunch is an important meal, but chances are, it is also the most unpredictable meal of the day. Your routine could vary on a weekly basis or even change day to day. On a given day, you might not know where you are having lunch, or what you plan to have.

Keeping in mind the erratic nature of most dieters' lunch schedules, I have devised flexible COUNTDOWN options to make life easier for you. First, the good news. Unlike dinner, you tend to work off your lunch calories through the day. This should therefore be your mainstay meal. But. (Sorry, but there's always a but!) But the bad news is too much food at lunch is going to make you lethargic and sleepy in the afternoon, because at this hour, the body's natural clock signals nap time.

You have to try to find a happy balance, like I did. When I'm working, I prefer a light lunch. With friends, lunch is a more elaborate affair, but I'm still watching the calories.

WHAT DOES WEEK 4 HAVE IN STORE?

This is the final week of your FOUR-WEEK COUNTDOWN, a week when your entire diet plan gets activated. For the first time, you will be eating as per the COUNTDOWN guidelines through the entire day. The transition is so gradual that this final lap of your COUNTDOWN should continue to be smooth and seamless.

The best part about week 4? This is the time you start seeing results. Your weight should be down a few notches on the scale . . . giving you every reason to cheer!

As with your other COUNTDOWN menus, lunch also provides balanced nutrition, the 1, 2, 3 Formula, that includes the 3 basic food groups.

1. CEREALS provide the carbs your body needs for energy.
2. FRUITS & VEGETABLES are nature's providers of vitamins, minerals & fibre.
3. PROTEIN-RICH FOODS are required for body repair and re-growth.

I hardly need to remind you that the success of your diet plan depends on how much you eat, and how often. As you know, the COUNTDOWN gears your system for more frequent meals, in smaller quantities. Again, your body will have adapted to this new eating technique and it is vital you continue with this routine even after the 4 weeks of your COUNTDOWN are complete.

For full details on how to proceed after the FOUR-WEEK COUNTDOWN runs its course, please refer to the Way Forward chapter.

MEN NEED MORE CALORIES EVERY DAY

Men and women have different metabolic rates. Men, because they have more muscle tissue, burn more calories than women and must therefore consume an additional number of calories during the course of the day.

In week 4 of the COUNTDOWN, men must add:

1 SERVING CEREAL + 1 SERVING PROTEIN-RICH FOOD
This extra allowance can be consumed during breakfast, lunch, or in-betweens.

LUNCH CHECK-IN

Choose your lunch based on how much weight you need to lose. Please refer to my Plan Minimum, Plan Medium and Plan Maximum to slot yourself correctly.

Check your Daily Food Guide in Annexure B to understand 'What makes one serving?' This determines the serving size of cereal, fruit and veggie and protein-rich foods allowed for your particular Plan.

For more clarifications and options, please refer to Annexure B.

PLAN MINIMUM lunch
for women to lose up to 4 kilos

1 CEREAL 1 serving

2 small phulkas/1 large roti/1 large slice bread (made of any cereal)
or
1 katori cooked cereal of your choice (rice, pasta, poha, rawa)

+

2 FRUIT & VEGETABLE 2 servings

2 katoris of your choice (restrict potato, jackfruit, yam, banana)

+

3 PROTEIN-RICH FOOD 1 serving

1 katori moong dal or sprouts
or
4 cubes low-fat paneer/low-fat feta cheese/tofu/1 katori low-fat curd
or
1 medium-sized piece white meat (chicken breast/turkey breast/fish)
or
2 egg whites

PLAN MEDIUM lunch

for men to lose up to 4 kilos: for women to lose 5–10 kilos

1 CEREAL 1 serving

2 small phulkas/1 large roti/1 large slice bread (made of any cereal)
or
1 katori cooked cereal of your choice (rice, pasta, poha, rawa)
+

2 FRUIT & VEGETABLE 2 servings

2 katoris of your choice (restrict potato, jackfruit, yam, banana, mango)
+

3 PROTEIN-RICH FOOD 1 serving

1 katori moong dal or sprouts
or
4 cubes low-fat paneer/low-fat feta cheese/tofu/1 katori low-fat curd

or
1 medium-sized piece white meat (chicken breast/turkey breast/fish)
or
2 egg whites

PLAN MAXIMUM lunch

for men to lose more than 5 kilos: for women to lose more than 11 kilos

1 CEREAL 2 servings

2 large rotis/2 large slices bread (made of any cereal)
or
2 katoris cooked cereal of your choice (rice, pasta, poha, rawa)

+

2 FRUIT & VEGETABLE 2 servings

2 katoris of your choice (restrict potato, jackfruit, yam, banana)

+

3 PROTEIN-RICH FOOD 1 serving

1 katori moong dal or sprouts
or
4 cubes low-fat paneer/low-fat feta cheese/tofu/1 katori low-fat curd
or
1 medium-sized piece white meat (chicken breast/turkey breast/fish)
or
2 egg whites

FACT FILE

Men have more testosterone than women. Testosterone is a hormone that promotes the development of muscle. Therefore a man's more muscular body burns more calories at rest and during exercise.

BUFFET LUNCH

When you attend a buffet, make a conscious effort not to succumb to temptation! Learn to eat smart. Pick the items that you are allowed. Most importantly, stay within your limit. Go for the salads, but avoid creamy dressings. Choose healthy options for your protein pick. And have cereals that do not come saturated with fat. Choose tandoori roti over the paratha, or stay with plain rice instead of helping yourself to rich pulao.

I have a little trick here that I'd like to share. I help myself generously to the vegetables and salads, so that my plate looks like I'm not on a diet. But, of course, I am fully aware that I am on a diet, and I stick to low-cal options. That way, I eat guilt-free.

LUNCH ON THE GO

A portable lunch is quick and easy to prepare. Wraps, rolls, and sandwiches are all convenient options.

Keep in mind, whatever option you choose, include your 1,2,3 Formula. For example, if you opt for a sandwich, and you have a single bread slice allowance, make it an open sandwich. Spread your ½ teaspoon quota of butter over the slice of bread, top it with slices of tomato and cucumber. Add a milky decaf coffee accompaniment and your 3 basic food groups are complete.

bread slice—cereal
sliced veggies—veggie
milky decaf coffee—protein-rich food

Non-vegetarians can carry a chicken sandwich, along with an apple as their fruit/veggie option.

bread slice—cereal
apple—fruit
chicken—protein-rich food

3-In-1 LUNCH OPTIONS

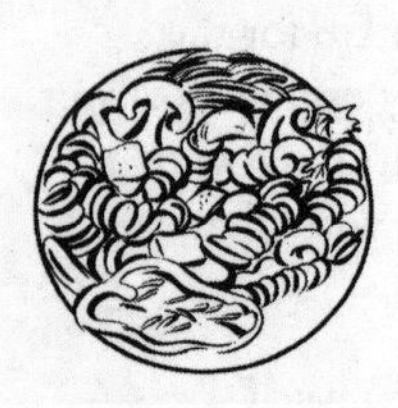

One-dish lunches are another delicious variation. Very popular in Oriental cuisines, Thai, Chinese, or Vietnamese fare offers some really delicious one-dish menus. Great low-calorie choices include warm broth with noodles and veggies plus tofu or chicken.

noodles—cereal
veggies—veggie
tofu or paneer or chicken—protein-rich food

When I want a working lunch, I often enjoy a Greek salad with a slice of bread. It's light and easy to make, and what's more I get to have my favourite feta cheese! In summer particularly, I find this a very refreshing lunch menu that also takes care of my 1,2,3 requirements. Once I get the salad ready, I drizzle a little balsamic vinegar and a few drops of extra virgin olive oil over it—and I'm good to go.

bread slice—cereal
romaine lettuce leaves, olives—veggie
low-fat feta cheese—protein-rich food

THE CASE OF THE TRAVELLING SALESMAN

Mr Nadkar was a travel company representative selling holiday packages. He often had to keep to tight schedules and manage his lunch in between appointments. He disliked eating in restaurants, so his wife usually packed a dabba, which he carried on his scooter.

In an attempt to please him, his wife generously added oil and ghee to the food, putting in her best efforts to prepare varied and delicious menus. In time, all those extra heavy lunches made Mr Nadkar put on weight. He developed a sizeable paunch. Not just that, he felt extra sleepy in the afternoon! So, with the help of a doctor friend, he decided to re-vamp his lunch. He was advised to eat light, but also pack proper nutrition into his portable meal. The doctor advised a balanced lunch, containing carbs, vitamins and minerals, and proteins. Mrs Nadkar, ever resourceful, used her ingenuity to prepare meals that were enjoyable, light and balanced. She found innovative ways to meet her husband's requirements.

Mr Nadkar loved his roti and veggie wrap (cereal and vegetable) with 1 cup curd (protein). He occasionally enjoyed a paneer tikka roll (cereal and protein) with kachumbar (veggie.) In the hot summer months he relished his favourite dahi bhaat with diced cucumber and tomato (cereal, protein and vegetable) all mixed together and packed in a thermoware container.

The experiment, overall, was extremely successful. Mr Nadkar not only lost the extra kilos but was much more alert through the day. He continued to enjoy home-cooked meals and was proud of his wife's cooking abilities. Instead of nodding off after a heavy lunch, he was all revved up, to make his next deal.

QUICK RECAP

- Eat small quantities at regular intervals, to balance your blood sugar.
- Plan and prepare your healthy meals in advance, then stick to them.
- Maintain a weekly food diary, making a note of your weak spots.

- Discard food 'triggers' such as fast-food takeaway leaflets.
- Drink more water, you may find you are thirsty rather than hungry!
- Mentally place yourself as a 'healthy eater'.
- Use herbs and spices to add zing to your food.

LUNCH RECIPES

1 katori = ½ cup = 100 grams
2 katoris = 1 cup = 200 grams

Lunch serving suggestions given here are for Plan Minimum and Plan Medium. If you are following Plan Maximum, just double the cereal portion, and retain the same serving sizes for the rest of the menu.

1, 2, 3 LUNCH COMBO SUGGESTIONS

1 katori (½ cup) rice + 2 katoris (1 cup) kachumbar + 1 serving tomato fish
or
1 slice whole-wheat bread + 2 katoris (1 cup) sautéed mushrooms + 1 serving chicken a la king
or
1 roti + 2 katoris (1 cup) mixed vegetable sabzi + 2 katoris (1 cup) mint-yoghurt raita
or
1 katori (½ cup) brown rice + 2 katoris (1 cup) green vegetable + 1 katori (½ cup) yellow moong dal
or
1 katori (½ cup) garlic-paneer noodles + 2 katoris (1 cup) steamed veggies
or
1 tandoori roti + 2 katoris (1 cup) okra vegetable + 1 katori green moong dal

TOMATO FISH 4 servings

Ingredients

4 medium-sized pieces fish fillet (any firm white fish)
2 onions, finely chopped
1 green capsicum, cut into julienne strips
2 green chillis, slit vertically
2 inch piece ginger, cut into julienne strips
handful mint leaves, chopped
salt to taste

Ingredients for the sauce

1 onion, chopped fine
4 tomatoes, chopped fine
4 cloves garlic, crushed
1 teaspoon chilli powder
1 tablespoon arrowroot powder
1 katori water
2 tablespoons wine vinegar
pinch sugar
1 teaspoon oil
salt to taste

Method for the sauce

To make the sauce, simmer the tomatoes, onion, garlic, salt and chili powder together for 20 minutes. Sieve the sauce and discard the tomato skins, then return the sauce to a clean pan. Heat the pan again, stir the sauce.

Mix the arrowroot and water to a smooth paste, then add it to the tomato sauce, along with the wine vinegar and sugar, stirring continuously till the sauce thickens.

Method for the fish

Heat the oil and fry the chopped onions and until soft. Remove onions from the pan and set aside. Add the fish and salt to the same oil and brown the fish on gently on both sides. Return the onions to the pan along with the slit green chillies, ginger and capsicum. Pour the tomato sauce over the fish pieces.

Cook the fish for about 5 minutes then take pan off the fire. Garnish with mint leaves. Serve hot, with the rice and kachumbar suggestion.

CHICKEN A LA KING 4 servings

Ingredients

2 chicken breasts, cooked, and cut into bite size pieces
½ teaspoon olive oil
1 onion chopped
1 green pepper, seeded and chopped
2–3 pods garlic crushed
1 teaspoon ground nutmeg
salt & pepper to taste

Method

Heat oil and sauté onion, green, peppers and garlic. Add the cooked chicken and seasoning. Serve hot, with a slice of multigrain bread.

MIXED VEGETABLE SUBZI 4 servings 4 katoris (2 cups)

Ajwain, also known as carom seeds, gives this vegetable its unique Mediterranean flavour.

Ingredients

1 katori carrots, cut lengthwise
1 katori beans, cut lengthwise
1 katori brinjal cut into 1 inch pieces
1 katori onions, sliced lengthwise
1 katori tomatoes, sliced lengthwise
1 teaspoon ajwain seeds
½ teaspoon garam masala
½ teaspoon turmeric powder
¼ teaspoon chilli powder
1 teaspoon oil
salt to taste

Method

Heat the oil in a frying pan (or non-stick pan), add ajwain seeds and onions. Sauté until onions are transparent.

Add the carrots and beans, sauté for 5 minutes. Then add the brinjal and sauté until all the vegetables are cooked tender. Add turmeric powder, tomatoes, garam masala, chilli powder, and salt, sauté for a few minutes until the tomatoes are tender, but not completely pulpy.

Leaving the tomatoes half-cooked adds to the fresh flavour. Serve hot. Please note the 5 katoris of vegetables will become 4 katoris when cooked.

GREEN VEGETABLE 4 servings 2 katoris (1 cup)

Ingredients

2 large bunches fresh mustard greens (sarson ka saag)
1 large bunch spinach
1 teaspoon ginger-garlic paste
4 green chillis, sliced
1 teaspoon lemon juice
a pinch garam masala
salt to taste

Ingredients for the tempering

1 teaspoon mustard oil
1 onion grated
a pinch red chili powder
a pinch of asafoetida (hing)

Method

Clean and wash the sarson and spinach thoroughly. Chop leaves and tender stems. Pressure cook the sarson, spinach, ginger-garlic paste and a pinch of salt in about 1 katori water. Keep on a low flame for 3–4 minutes. Cool the vegetable and grind into a thick puree.

Heat mustard oil in a non-stick pan and add asafoetida, saute onions until done. Pour in the pureed greens, allow to sizzle in the hot oil. Add the red chilli powder and lemon juice. Serve hot.

GARLIC-PANEER NOODLES 4 servings

Ingredients

4 katoris boiled cooked noodles (whole wheat)
2 stalks celery, diagonally sliced
1 white onion, sliced
4 cloves garlic, minced
1 teaspoon hot chilli sauce
1 teaspoon light soya sauce
1 teaspoon white vinegar
16 cubes low-fat paneer cubes, of 1 inch x 1 inch size (4 cubes per serving)
1 teaspoon sesame oil

Method

Heat oil to high heat in wok or deep skillet. Add onion, celery, garlic and cook, stirring often, for 3 to 5 minutes. Add paneer, soy sauce, hot sauce, vinegar. Immerse the noodles in boiling salted water for 1 minute, or until tender.

Drain noodles and toss into the wok, mix well. Serve hot.

OKRA (LADIES FINGER) VEGETABLE 4 servings 4 katoris (2 cups)

Ingredients
4 katoris okra, washed and dried

Ingredients for the filling
2 tablespoons finely grated cabbage
½ teaspoon turmeric
¼ teaspoon red chili powder
a pinch of coriander powder (dhania)
1 teaspoon oil
salt to taste

Method
Slit the okra vertically, keep aside. Mix the remaining ingredients, and stuff as filling into the okra cavities. Brush the okra with 1 teaspoon of oil. Steam in a steamer, or place in a sieve, over a pot of boiling water. Cook till the okra wilts, and is no longer crunchy. Serve hot.

SECTION II

THE WAY FORWARD

CHAPTER 12

WEEK 5 ONWARDS

THE CASE OF THE YO-YO DIETER

A client of mine, Smita Kothari, is an NRI who lives in the US. She has a hectic, jet-set lifestyle with very little time to follow any fixed diet. So whenever she was abroad, Smita would always read the food labels and regulate her eating. Very often, to lose weight 'fast' she would starve, or just nibble salad greens.

But then, the urge to enjoy the occasional cocktail, or indulge in an all-you-can-eat buffet was always very tempting. At first, Smita would try to control these cravings. But then, her social life was demanding. Irregular hours and regular partying came with a price. So Smita would go all-out, gorging on the fancy cocktail snacks and gourmet dinners.

When her designer jeans got a little too snug and subsequently, impossible to even zip up, Smita would do some soul-searching. Remorseful and desperate to make amends, she would then swing towards the other extreme, resorting to diet protein shakes and salad greens. This often made her sick and very often, hungry and irritable too. So once again there would be another phase of out-of-control bingeing. And so it went on.

Of course, Smita needed help, and fast. When she came to me, she was in one of her starving phases. I convinced her to try a balanced diet plan, with small frequent meals. She did not think it would work and told me so! I persuaded her to just trust me, and give me 4 weeks of her time.

I saw Smita exactly 4 weeks later. She could not believe her own transformation. Her skin glowed, her eyes shone, she looked trim and fit. While she had some more weight to lose, Smita was well on her way to a steady, safe weight-loss regimen.

Now, I see her featured in the society columns from time to time, always looking stunning in her haute couture creations. Clearly, Smita has discovered her way forward.

Congratulations on making the four-week mark!

I am sure you have accomplished a lot during your FOUR-WEEK COUNTDOWN. Your hard work is showing and you are, without a doubt, feeling good about yourself.

At this point, you are on the threshold of a completely new way of life, at a crucial juncture in your fight against flab. Poor food habits have been modified, excesses eliminated.

A word of caution here. It's very easy to slip back into the comfort zone of your old routine. So be prepared to fight the urge! Now is not the time to lose your hard-earned advantage and let it all go. This happens to dieters more often than you can imagine.

Once the initial euphoria of losing weight wears off, your willpower tends to wear down too. Many dieters feel the need for a 'release' and start bingeing like there's no tomorrow. But of course, as we all know, there is a tomorrow. And a day after. And a week after that. What is important is to take each day as it comes. Some of you will be near your target weight loss goal. Many will have more weight to

lose. Either way, you will have to continue to be vigilant about your diet and exercise routine.

All my clients hope to get off the 'diet' and get back to 'normal'. I hate to break it to you, but normal no longer means fried goodies and all-you-can-eat indulgences, and never will!

You must continue to eat sensibly, in moderation, and make sure you eat balanced meals that include the 1,2,3 Formula. That is the 'new normal', a lifestyle change you have to embrace in the long run.

Focus on long-term changes related to your diet and physical activity. Keep reminding yourself that, if you revert to your old eating habits, the weight is going to bounce back.

Moreover, external pressures, such as media messages promising magical solutions, or dieters who resort to drastic measures for weight loss, are influences you should beware of. 'How to be even skinnier' is a false promise that lures you into feeling dissatisfied. Don't fall victim to the hype. Take comfort in the fact that you are working towards your ideal weight and building a healthy lifestyle that fits in with who you are.

In fact, I would suggest, don't even call your routine a 'diet' any more. Because a diet is temporary and what you are looking at is a permanent change. To get yourself on track for long-term success just build your dietary plan into your lifestyle. It is no longer a diet, but a way of life.

FACT FILE

Many dieters find 'before and after' photographs work. It is a great way to remind yourself of the progress you have made!

Week 5 to week 8

The FOUR-WEEK COUNTDOWN helps to gradually ease you into a diet. By week 5, your routine is well set and, as you persevere, the weight will continue to melt away. During the initial four-week period, your weight loss was mainly restricted to carbohydrate weight loss and water loss per kilo, rather than an actual decrease in body fat. But now, from week 5 onwards, your body is physically primed for greater fat loss in percentage terms. Make the most of it!

Beyond the FOUR-WEEK COUNTDOWN, up to week 9, your Diet Plan must match your weight loss goals. Choose Plan Minimum, Plan Medium, or Plan Maximum, as per your requirements. Please note that in all the Diet Plans, calorie-counting is already factored in, but your food intake is not based on calories alone, it's based on optimal nutrition choices.

From week 9 onwards, you can start with the Way Forward. During your Way Forward, you will once again slot yourself into Plan Minimum, Plan Medium or Plan Maximum, based on weight loss requirements. Please refer to the following pages to find your Way Forward.

PLAN MINIMUM way forward
For women to lose up to 4 kilos

BREAKFAST

Bonus allowance 1 cup tea/coffee

1 serving cereal
+
1 serving fruit/vegetable
+
1 serving protein-rich food

LUNCH

1 serving cereal
+
2 servings fruit/vegetable
+
1 serving protein-rich food

IN-BETWEENS

Mid morning In-Between	beverage + *bite	(cereal)
Afternoon In-Between	beverage + *bite	(fruit/vegetable)
Evening In-Between	beverage + *bite	(protein-rich food)

*bites can be interchanged

DINNER

Starter Sip unlimited
+
Nutri Bowl 1 cup
+
Fibre Filler 1 cup
+
1, 2, 3 Main Course Dinner

½ serving cereal
+
1 serving vegetable
+
1 serving protein-rich food

PLAN MEDIUM way forward

for men to lose up to 4 kilos : for women to lose 5–10 kilos

Note: MEN NEED MORE CALORIES EVERY DAY

1 SERVING CEREAL + 1 SERVING PROTEIN-RICH FOOD

This extra allowance can be consumed during breakfast, lunch, or in-betweens.

BREAKFAST: Bonus allowance 1 cup tea/coffee

2 servings cereal
+
1 serving fruit or vegetable
+
1 serving protein-rich food

LUNCH

1 serving cereal
+
2 servings fruit/vegetable
+
1 serving protein-rich food

IN-BETWEENS

Mid morning In-Between	beverage + *bite	(cereal)
Afternoon In-Between	beverage + *bite	(fruit/vegetable)
Evening In-Between	beverage + *bite	(protein-rich food)

*bites can be interchanged

DINNER

Starter Sip unlimited
+
Nutri Bowl 1 cup
+
Fibre Filler 1 cup
+
1, 2, 3 Main Course Dinner

1 serving cereal
+
1 serving vegetable
+
1 serving protein-rich food

PLAN MAXIMUM way forward

For men to lose more than 5 kilos or For women to lose more than 11 kilos

Note: MEN NEED MORE CALORIES EVERY DAY

1 SERVING CEREAL + 1 SERVING PROTEIN-RICH FOOD

This extra allowance can be consumed during breakfast, lunch, or in-betweens.

BREAKFAST: Bonus allowance 1 cup tea/coffee

2 servings cereal
+
1 serving fruit or vegetable
+
1 serving protein-rich food

LUNCH

2 servings cereal
+
2 servings fruit/vegetable
+
1 serving protein-rich food

IN-BETWEENS

Mid morning In-Between	beverage + *bite	(cereal)
Afternoon In-Between	beverage + *bite	(fruit/vegetable)
Evening In-Between	beverage + *bite	(protein-rich food)

DINNER

Starter Sip unlimited
+
Nutri Bowl 1 cup
+
Fibre Filler 1 cup
+
1, 2, 3 Main Course Dinner

1 serving cereal
+
1 serving vegetable
+
2 servings protein-rich food

Week 9 onwards

I have anticipated some questions that would come up regarding the Way Forward. The answers here help to guide you into your new phase.

Q. I have reached my optimum weight; how long do I stay on the diet?

A. Re-visit the word 'diet' and re-look at your new eating habits. Make the changes a way of life. Most people put on weight after dieting because they get back to their old eating habits, resulting in weight gain.

FACT FILE

Research has proved that it takes time to adjust to reduced weight. It takes one year for your body to fully stabilize at the new weight level.

Q. What do I do if I need to lose more weight after the 8-week period?

A. At week 9, re-assess your weight loss goals or check your BMI. If it is lower than before, switch to the appropriate Diet Plan. If it is the same as before, stay with the same Plan.

For example, if you were on **Plan Maximum**, and your weight has reduced, you may need to shift to **Plan Medium** from week 9, in order to ensure further weight loss.

Q. I need to lose weight fast. Can I shift from Plan Maximum to Plan Minimum?

A. Do not make the mistake of going on a drastic diet! Cutting calories gradually is the smartest way of losing weight and keeping it off. Believe it or not, you may not see the results you want to see because you are not eating enough. If you slash your calories to abnormal levels, your body perceives this as a starvation threat. As a result, your body metabolism slows down. This is what happens to drastic dieters:

1. Your body gets used to less food and to continue losing weight, and you will need to keep decreasing your food intake.
2. You lose muscle mass and therefore decrease your metabolic rate.
3. You may be at risk of health problems, as inadequate nutrition leads to weakness and lowers immune system responses.
4. It is virtually impossible to stay on a low-cal diet for prolonged periods.
5. Drastic dieters have high dropout rates, simply because the changes are so radical.

Q. I'm a smoker. If I give up smoking, I know I'll bloat up. Help!

A. True, the nicotine in cigarettes works as an appetite suppressant. But it also kills your taste buds, increases the pressure on your heart, and ruins your lungs. Do you really want that?

Quite apart from the internal damage are problems like premature facial wrinkles, bad breath and discoloured teeth. These are just some of the negatives. In fact, the risks are so numerous and the consequences so detrimental to your health, that it would be completely foolhardy to continue smoking only to lose weight.

Q. What happens when I slip up?

A. Read the chapter on diet slip-ups to understand that an occasional indulgence is no deterrent to long-term goals.

Q. Can I stop exercising once I lose weight?

A. Exercise should be a part of your daily life. It keeps your weight in check and helps avoid a relapse into sedentary lifestyle patterns.

Q. I am off on vacation, and I'm not sure I can keep my COUNTDOWN going. Where do I start when I return from my trip?

A. You could start from day 1 of the FOUR-WEEK COUNTDOWN. Alternatively, if you have completed the entire COUNTDOWN, and are ready for week 5, you could move on to the Way Forward.

Q. There are times when I don't feel like staying with the 1, 2, 3 Formula. For example, I want to skip the veggies. Will I still lose weight?

A. Don't knock the veggies; they are there for a very good reason! If you omit veggies as a one-off example, it's okay. But remember, once you get into the habit of eating balanced meals and your body gets adequate nutrition, you actually start feeling much fitter and healthier. So if you deprive yourself of the 1, 2, 3 Formula, your body craves good nourishment again, tempting you to turn to quick-fix foods, such as sugar. That defeats the very purpose of your diet.

HOW MY SNACKING WENT FROM FRIED TO ROASTED

While we are on the subject, I should tell you how much trouble I had, keeping to a sustained food plan. I loved the idea of snacks with my chai, snacks with my friends, snacks with anything I did! So, for me, it was torture having to turn down home-made puris and kachoris, or say no to my favorite butter biscuits and nankhatai.

But because I love these treats so much, I look for substitutes. Have you tried Marie biscuits with a bit of peanut butter? Or toast with a green coriander chutney spread? I love a good bhel too, with sprouted moong, chaat masala, tamarind chutney and onion! The point is, don't feel sorry for yourself, just because you are giving up the grease. Let your imagination run riot and you will be amazed at the ideas you can cook up.

Now, in fact, I find the deep fried stuff hard to handle, They seem too heavy and far too oily for my taste. Today, my palate has evolved to enjoy lighter fare, a transition that has happened over a period of time. Eating right has become my new way of life.

THE CASE OF THE PLATEAUING DIETER

When your weight loss comes to a standstill, even though you continue with your diet and exercise regimen, it can be very disheartening. Sonu Pathak, a student of mine, was a classic example. He lost 2 kilos in one month. But after that, although Sonu continued his diet, his weight refused to budge.

Sonu's could have been a case of the diet plateau, where his body had adjusted to the reduced calories, so he just stopped losing weight. Alternately, it could be an exercise plateau problem, in which his body has accounted for his exercise-burning calories, and was no longer responding to the extra stimulus!

There is no scientific method to tell you exactly where the problem lies. Therefore, to break out of a plateau, it is necessary to reduce calorie intake and step up exercise. Also keep in mind, if you are nearer your ideal weight level, as Sonu was, it is always tougher to shed the remaining kilos.

So how did Sonu outsmart his body and break out of the plateau?

1. The trick is, never be predictable, because the body learns to adjust to routine. It helps to vary the type of exercise or

regime every 6 weeks, so that different muscles are constantly challenged.

2. Once a week, say every Thursday, I suggest a dinner of fruit and skimmed milk, or a soup and salad meal, again, to break the routine.

Sonu incorporated both these changes into his fitness programme, and sure enough, he was back on track towards his weight loss goals.

It's easy to be lazy.

I'd like to add something at this point. Do not, please, do not compare yourself with others. Every one is made differently. So it stands to reason that everybody will lose weight differently. There is no point getting depressed if someone you know is losing weight faster than you are! Some people just have to work a little harder than others to lose weight.

So find something that works for you. Keep your goal in sight, and do whatever you have to do to meet that goal. I admit, it's not easy. Often, I get lazy and lose sight of these goals myself. But I make it a point to keep track of my daily activities and watch my weight. I pick myself up and get going once again, on the Way Forward!

QUICK RECAP

- Don't skip meals. Continue to eat 6 balanced, low-fat meals.
- Sit down to eat your meals, chew well, take time over your food and pay attention to what you eat.
- Slot exercise in your daily planner.
- Keep up self-monitoring by weighing in once a week. Unless you know what your weight is, you can't keep it in check.
- Don't wait till your weight increases from 1 kilo to 5 kilos—do something about it right away.
- Think lifestyle change rather than sticking with the diet mentality.
- Find new and exciting ways to stay motivated.

- Reward yourself for reaching small weight loss goals.
- Connect with friends and ask for support. If you are online, connect with like-minded groups.
- Continue to set realistic weight loss targets, turn small goals into bigger goals.
- Keep a journal of your food consumption—it helps you stay on track.

CHAPTER 13

DRINKING & DIETING

I hate to break this to you but very simply put, drinking and dieting don't mix!

You have probably heard that one before. But if you are a regular one-drink-an-evening person, it might be hard to completely give up the alcohol. While abstaining is definitely the preferred option, at the risk of sounding repetitive, I will reiterate once again: the COUNTDOWN, as always, is flexible!

Indulge in that occasional drink if you must, without going overboard. I don't drink myself; however, most of my friends do. Indeed, the trend towards alcohol consumption appears to have increased, both among men and women. Keeping this in mind, I concluded it would be easier to go with the flow rather than ban alcohol completely, because chances are you are going to drink anyway.

Most often, I find the consumption of alcohol is an evening phenomenon, in the company of friends or business associates, or a pre-dinner drink when 'unwinding' at home. I have therefore addressed dinner-time drinking in this chapter. I am giving you the option of having that occasional drink without ruining your diet. But please do LIMIT your consumption, otherwise you will not get the weight loss results you desire.

Once you get a sense of how calorie-dense alcohol actually is, the figures will really make you sit up. Some of you may even voluntarily decide to give it a miss, at least while your COUNTDOWN is on!

Alcoholic beverages are high in calories and, at 7 calories per gram of alcohol, are almost on par with fats! It is therefore critical to restrict your alcohol intake. Moreover, alcohol does not provide any nutrients, only empty calories.

Not all alcoholic beverages have the same alcohol content. If you have a drink containing a higher-than-average percentage of alcohol, and mix the alcohol with beverages such as sweetened soft drinks, fruit juice or cream, you increase the number of total calories consumed. Did you know, for example, an innocuous Piña Colada packs in more than 250 calories? And that's not counting all the fried snacks you might consume along with it.

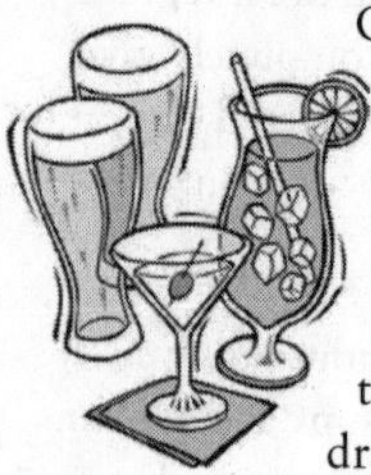

With the consumption of alcohol, your COUNTDOWN Dinner plan has to be modified, to budget for the extra calories you consume while drinking.

Cheers!

When you choose to have a drink during the COUNTDOWN, you don't have to worry about counting calories. I have already done an extensive study, where I have listed out various alcohol options, with recommended serving sizes. Each of these units adds up to the same number of calories, approximately 130 calories each, so regardless of what you drink, the calorie count remains constant.

This means no one drink is 'better' or 'worse' in terms of calories consumed—all have equal calorific value.

A wide selection of alcoholic beverages are listed here, along with a recommended unit allowance. Go with the drink of your choice but remember to stick to the RECOMMENDED UNIT ALLOWANCE ONLY.

The following table is a guide to the quantity of alcohol permissible during your COUNTDOWN. Unit sizes are mentioned—in terms of can, peg, glass, or shot—use these standard units to measure your particular drink.

CHOOSE ANY ONE DRINK FROM THIS LIST

BEER

Beer regular 330 ml	allowance: 1 can
Beer light 330 ml	allowance: 1 & ½ cans

DISTILLED SPIRIT

Rum	allowance: 2 small pegs 30 ml each or 1 large peg 60 ml
Whiskey	allowance: 2 small pegs 30 ml each or 1 large peg 60 ml
Scotch	allowance: 2 small pegs 30 ml each or 1 large peg 60 ml
Vodka	allowance: 2 small pegs 30 ml each or 1 large peg 60 ml
Gin	allowance: 2 small pegs 30 ml each or 1 large peg 60 ml

TABLE WINE

Dry White Wine	allowance: 1½ glasses @ 120 ml per glass	180 ml total
Red/Rose Wine	allowance: 1½ glasses @ 120 ml per glass	180 ml total
Sweet Wine	allowance: ¾ glass @ 120 ml per glass	90 ml total

SPARKLING WINE

Champagne	allowance: 1 ¼ glass @ 120 ml per glass	150 ml total

OTHERS

Any liqueur	allowance: 1 small peg	30 ml total
Tequila	allowance: 2 shots	120 ml total
Brandy/Cognac	allowance: 1 ½ pegs	45 ml total

STANDARD MEASURE CHART FOR DISTILLED SPIRITS

RUM }	
WHISKY }	
VODKA }	1 small peg 30 ml
GIN }	1 large peg 60 ml
BRANDY }	
COGNAC }	

STANDARD MEASURE CHART FOR 1 GLASS OF WINE

WHITE WINE }	
RED WINE }	
ROSE }	range from 120–150 ml
SWEET WINE }	
CHAMPAGNE }	

TEQUILA SHOT 60 ml

LIQUEURS 30 ml (mostly)

NOTE: The standard measure for 1 glass of wine ranges from 120 ml to 150 ml, depending on the restaurant where it is served. Wine glasses may also vary slightly in size. For your reference and for the purpose of the COUNTDOWN, I have used a 120 ml glass as a standard measure.

LOW CAL NON-ALCOHOLIC MIXERS

Club Soda
Sugar-Free Tonic
Fresh Lime Water
Diet Cola
Ice

TIPPLING TIPS

1. Dilute your drink with soda.
2. Add ice cubes to keep it light and chilled.
3. Sip your drink slowly instead of guzzling it down.
4. Add a refreshing twist of sprigs of mint or a celery stick stirrer.
5. Alcohol dehydrates. Drink plenty of water before you start drinking. The thumb rule is: consume 1 glass of water for every serving of alcohol.
6. Dry red wines and white wines are lower in calories than sweet dessert wines.
7. Munch low-cal snacks with your drink. Options such as unbuttered popcorn, roasted chips or julienne-cut crudités like carrots, cucumber or celery sticks make perfect accompaniments. Please keep in mind that your snacks count as part of dinner and must therefore be included as your dinner allowance.

SMOKING

Many drinkers I know love to light up and enjoy a smoke along with their drink. I certainly can't try to stop you from smoking, but you do know how lethal the habit is! Try to control the urge, by taking in and releasing your breath slowly, 5 times. This relaxes and calms your mind and may help to reduce the need to light up.

DINNER DIET PLAN WITH ALCOHOL

When you consume alcohol, you cannot follow the regular COUNTDOWN Diet Plan. You have to go with a revised dinner plan that balances your calorie intake and factors in the extra calories you have consumed. This way, even though you indulge in the occasional drink, you are still able to effectively maintain your weight-loss programme.

Please select your revised diet dinner with alcohol based on how much weight you need to lose. Refer to my Plan Minimum, Plan Medium and Plan Maximum to slot yourself correctly.

Check your Daily Food Guide in Annexure B to understand 'What makes one serving?' This determines the serving size of cereal, fruit and veggie and protein-rich foods allowed for your particular Plan.

For more clarifications and options, please refer to Annexure B.

PLAN MINIMUM with alcohol

for women to lose up to 4 kilos

DINNER FORMULA with alcohol

1. Fibre Filler
2. 1, 2, 3 Main Course as given below

1 CEREAL ½ serving

1 small phulka or 1 small slice bread (made of any cereal)
or
½ katori cooked cereal of your choice (rice, pasta, poha, rawa)

+

2 FRUIT & VEGETABLE 1 serving

1 katori of your choice (restrict potato, jackfruit, yam, banana)

+

3 PROTEIN-RICH FOOD 1 serving

1 katori moong dal or sprouts
or
4 cubes low-fat paneer/feta cheese/tofu/1 katori low-fat curd
or
1 medium-sized piece white meat (chicken/turkey breast or fish)
or
2 egg whites

PLAN MEDIUM with alcohol

For men to lose up to 4 kilos or women to lose 5–10 kilos

DINNER FORMULA with alcohol

1. Fibre Filler
2. 1, 2, 3 Main Course as given below

1 CEREAL 1 serving

2 small phulkas/1 large roti/1 large slice bread (made of any cereal)
or
1 katori cooked cereal of your choice (rice, pasta, poha, rawa)

+

2 FRUIT & VEGETABLE 1 serving

1 katori of your choice (restrict potato, jackfruit, yam, banana, mango)

+

3 PROTEIN-RICH FOOD 1 serving

1 katori moong dal or sprouts
or
4 cubes low-fat paneer/feta cheese/tofu/1 katori low-fat curd
or
1 medium-sized piece white meat (chicken/turkey breast or fish)
or
2 egg whites

PLAN MAXIMUM with alcohol
for men to lose more than 5 kilos or women to lose more than 11 kilos

DINNER FORMULA with alcohol

1. Fibre Filler
2. 1, 2, 3 Main Course as given below

1 CEREAL 1 serving

2 small phulkas/1 large roti/1 large slice bread (made of any cereal)
or

1 katori cooked cereal of your choice (rice, pasta, poha, rawa)

+

2 FRUIT & VEGETABLE 1 serving

1 katori of your choice (restrict potato, jackfruit, yam, banana)

+

3 PROTEIN-RICH FOOD 2 servings

2 katoris moong dal or sprouts
or
8 cubes low-fat paneer/feta cheese/tofu/2 katoris low-fat curd
or
2 medium-sized piece white meat (chicken/turkey breast or fish)
or
4 egg whites

HOW ALCOHOL PUTS THE BRAKES ON FAT LOSS

When you consume alcohol, your liver converts most of the alcohol into a substance called acetaldehyde. This is then converted into acetate and hydrogen. Your body uses the hydrogen in preference to fatty acids for its energy requirements, forcing the un-utilized fatty acids to get stored as fat. In addition, the chemical reaction may promote fatty acid synthesis, thereby increasing your accumulation of fat.

What does all this actually mean?

Your body doesn't burn its fuel on a first-come-first-serve basis. It has a fuel preference for alcohol! So when you drink, the alcohol gets burned off for energy before the fat gets a chance to start burning.

Think about it. The more you drink, the longer it will take you to lose weight. Imagine, after conscientiously sticking with your COUNTDOWN, only to lose out because you overdid the alcohol!

So make the smart choice, ration your alcohol, and keep your weight loss plan on track.

DON'T DRINK ON AN EMPTY STOMACH

There is a reason for it. Alcohol is an appetite stimulant, so if you drink on an empty stomach, you end up eating more for dinner. And don't forget, this is over and above all the snacks you have munched through while you were drinking!

THE CASE OF THE THWARTED BACHELOR

My student Karan Kumar is a young, upwardly mobile bachelor, who is highly conscious about fitness. He religiously works out at my classes at least 4 times a week. He regulates his food consumption and his meal-times. Yet, he came to me one day, surprised to find his weight increasing, particularly around the abdomen.

Karan could not understand why, in spite of his best efforts, he couldn't get the toned abs that he aspired to. Well, I was surprised too, until we went through Karan's schedule. I discovered he was a regular at his neighbourhood pub. That explained everything.

I helped Karan to make the connection between his alcohol intake and his expanding waistline. Like most men, Karan tended to expand around the abdominal region, because of increased activity of lipoprotein lipase in this area. Lipoprotein lipase is an enzyme that pushes triglycerides into the fat cells. Moreover, the liver starts metabolizing alcohol before it metabolizes fat, resulting in an increased storage of fat.

Karan figured he needed to cut back on the alcohol. After some serious introspection, he spared no effort to do so. His perseverance paid off. Today, he has the sculpted abs he desires and, from what I hear, quite a female following too!

CHAPTER 14

WHEN YOU SLIP OR GIVE UP

It's bound to happen. We are all human and there's no way anyone can maintain a perfect diet regimen day after day, week after week. There will be times when the temptation gets just too much. Don't be surprised if the overwhelming urge to binge breaks down your diet resolve. Or 'just one bite' turns into an eating orgy. Of course, when a couple of consecutive binges lead to an all-out meltdown, you know it's time to press the brakes, hard!

How do you handle the syndrome and what do you do?

Let me begin by saying you are no different from the millions of dieters who go through this. No one wants to give up their favourite dessert or stay away permanently from the fried goodies. It's normal to feel deprived, but hey, it's not the end of the world! If you learn to eat smart, you can still budget for occasional indulgences without breaking the bank, so to speak.

Always remember, dieting is progress, not perfection.
Perfectionists often fail as dieters because they inevitably fail to factor in natural slip-ups and eventually end up going off-diet. Will depriving yourself on a restrictive diet really help you lose

weight? Or will you end up binge-eating because you are craving the forbidden food?

Giving in occasionally is just fine. It works as an outlet for the frustration you sometimes feel. But I am here to help you lose weight. I cannot be of much help if you choose to let yourself go off course completely, because ultimately, you will hit a point of no return.

Let me share a little secret that usually works for me. Whenever I feel like indulging, I take a deep, deep breath. I shut my eyes and count up to 10. (Not necessarily aloud, especially if I'm out in public!) Then I think about something not connected to food that I particularly want. A new outfit? An Ipod? A haircut? A nice massage? A movie with a friend? I focus on this exciting new possibility. And 9 times out of 10, my urge to eat tapers off.

For that 1 in 10 chance, when the craving really builds up, I deal with the monster! I have learnt to manage slip-ups by working around them. If I indulge wisely, I know it's possible to stay on track. And instead of gaining weight, my metabolism adapts to the brief deviation.

FACT FILE

Fit and active people are better able to adjust extra calories than those who are sedentary. Another great reason to exercise!

Tip

Try and make wise choices, such as 'whole-grain', 'baked/grilled' 'low-fat' even when you indulge. In time, you may begin to prefer the healthier choices.

Unless you are superhuman, with unlimited willpower at your beck and call, I would take indulgences as a given. Like I said, it happens to everyone. So instead off curling up with guilt and going into alternate bingeing and starving phases, known as the 'yo-yo syndrome', it is much better to accept the fact that you will be tempted from time to time. Welcome to the real world!

That said, recognizing your weakness is key, because if you don't see the problem you can't solve it. So what is the solution? My answer may surprise you. **I'm categorically telling you, here and now: Please do not give up anything you really crave.**

CRAVE-O-METER CONTROL ON A SCALE OF 1 TO 10

Set yourself a CRAVE-O-METER to rate your cravings on a scale of 1 to 10. 1 is highest on your priority list, 10 not so important. What this helps you do is keep tabs on the 'not worth it' foods you consume.

1–2	3–4	5–6	7–8	9–10
I'll die without!	I must have at least one small bite	I can't seem to resist my carvings	I think I can say no this time	This is something I can safely pass up

So on a 1 to 10 scale, if a particular treat rates 8, it is pretty low down on your CRAVE-O-METER. But if something notches up 3, or 2, or 1, don't even try to resist!

Concentrate on indulging in the foods you really can't do without, the foods that rate 5 and up on your CRAVE-O-METER. Savour those foods slowly, enjoy every bite. While you indulge, forget the guilt. You owe yourself the occasional treat, because after this, you are back into your 'good' zone, leaving the happy memories behind!

After 4 weeks of your COUNTDOWN, you would have established regular eating and exercise habits. Now, how do you deal with temptation? After much research on the subject, I have developed two methods that work.

1. INDULGENCE **CONTROL:** Controlled indulgers need to maintain a check on their excesses, by planned consumption of foods they crave. Consciously indulge, but always in moderation.
2. BINGE-EATING **COMPENSATION:** Uncontrolled bingers must follow up with a compensation plan to make up for the extra consumption, by sticking to a modified, reduced-calorie dinner.

Indulgence control? Or binge eating?

Indulgence control may not work for everyone. Some people are just spontaneous eaters—bingeing is not something they plan! What describes you best? Given a choice, it is better to plan a meal of controlled indulgence rather than binge eating. Here are the reasons why.

- You are more in control of your eating, as opposed to bingeing, which can become an out-of-control excess.
- You get into the habit of portion control—a habit that will help you stop the cravings that result in an all-out eating binge.
- If you schedule weekly slips, you factor in the indulgence, and are far less likely to plunge into a spontaneous free fall.

Please keep in mind, whether you go for INDULGENCE CONTROL or BINGE-EATING COMPENSATION, the limits are set by you. This is an issue you must psychologically resolve with yourself. The real guilt of indulging comes from the belief that deviating from a perfect diet plan can negate all your hard work. But that is not the case. Your body responds to what you eat over time, not what you eat at one meal.

Both INDUGENCE CONTROL and BINGE-EATING COMPENSATION must be occasional, ideally not more than once a week. Try to further reduce the frequency to once in 2 weeks.

1. INDULGENCE CONTROL

Even controlled indulgence has its rules! When you indulge, moderation is the key. If you enjoy that occasional pizza, figure out what portion size you would normally consume. Cut your usual portion by half. Start your pizza lunch with a low-cal beverage. Follow it up with a bowl of fruit or salad. Then take the time to savour your half portion of pizza lunch. Sit and talk with a friend and enjoy your treat. Factor in this luxury as a weekly indulgence, if you wish. Enjoy it. And you'll do just fine.

RULE: Eat half of what you normally would indulge in. Doggie bag the rest or share it with someone who will enjoy it.

Controlled Indulgence: MEAL Formula

Beverage + Fibre Filler + Half portion of meal indulgence

Controlled Indulgence: IN-BETWEENS Formula

Beverage + Half portion snack indulgence

FIBRE FILLER 1 cup

FIBRE FILLERS consist of juicy veggies, fruits, crisp sprouts and crunchy salads. Add more zest to your FIBRE FILLER with a dash of lime juice, chaat masala or a bit of salt and pepper. Feel free to experiment.

1 cup veggie salad (tomato, cucumber, carrot, celery, lettuce)
or
1 cup fruit salad (orange, apple, sweet lime, pear, papaya)
or
1 cup fruit and veggie salad (apple, celery, lettuce, sweet lime)

CHOOSE YOUR BEVERAGE 1 CUP

skimmed milk
or
buttermilk
or
soup/rasam
or
vegetable juice
or
herbal tea or decaf tea or coffee
or
coconut water
or
coffee with ½ serving milk (1 katori) + 1 teaspoon sugar
or
plain tea/masala tea/cardamom tea/ginger tea
with ½ serving milk (1 katori) +1 teaspoon sugar

2. BINGE-EATING COMPENSATION

THE CASE OF THE BINGE EATER

Now we come to the case of the spontaneous binge eater. A perfect example was my client, Aditya Katrak. Being a party person, Aditya loved being out with friends. On nights out, he could eat his weight in steak, blowing his careful calorie counting through the day! The next morning, he would be remorseful, wishing he hadn't gone to town on that 'awesome' pub fare.

Instead of repenting, I told him it would be helpful if he stopped repeating the offence! I explained to Aditya, while it was okay to mess up occasionally, making it a habit was not going to help his cause. Aditya needed something that worked, for his way of life. I mean, I could see his point of view. When you are having fun with friends, calories are the last thing on your mind. But once you over-indulge, you have to make it up by cutting your calorie intake the next day. This is the only way to balance out the extra calories consumed.

Aditya heard me out and was fully prepared to atone for his sins, by compensating the next day! The guidelines I offered him are outlined here, for you. Like Aditya, you too can keep your weight in check by following my **Compensation Dinner Formula.**

If you deviate at breakfast or lunch, compensate the same day at dinner. If you deviate at dinner, compensate next day at dinner.

Compensation Dinner Formula

1. Starter Sip: unlimited
2. Nutri Bowl: unlimited
3. Fibre Filler: unlimited (exclude bananas, mangoes, chikoos and sitaphal)

AVOID MAIN COURSE

Your Compensation Dinner fills you up, without actually having the Main Course. You will consume a liquid, yet another thicker liquid (Nutri-Bowl), and the Fibre Filler, which works as a high water-content appetizer. While the quality and quantity of your food is important, you can eat to your satisfaction.

FACT FILE

Fruit and veggies are natural cleansers and make a great detox meal.

ASSOCIATING FOOD WITH A PARTICULAR PLACE

How often do you link a particular culinary specialty with a particular place? I always associate vada pav with Lonavala, or chocolate brownies with the Willingdon Club in Mumbai. I'm sure all of us have our favourite food spots, where we look forward to enjoying the very thing the place is famous for. Your taste could run to kebabs at Nizams in Delhi or a big dim sum spread at your favourite Chinese restaurant in Kolkata.

Whatever your preference, you would want to go out of your way to eat it! So if you are planning any such expedition, go prepared. It is better go reach your destination with a clear idea of what you plan to eat and the extent of your excesses.

CHAPTER 15

READ THE LABEL

In the frenetic pace of our daily routine, convenience foods help us keep our sanity! However, the mind-boggling variety of bottles, packets, polybags, tetra packs and foil trays that line the supermarket shelves can be quite daunting. How do you evaluate what you are getting? How do you compare one product with another? Let's try to read between the lines and make some smart choices.

International labels follow very strict guidelines. In India, laws are becoming more stringent, and brands are required to adhere to a code that meets government-approved packaged food requirements. As labels and brands become more accountable, it's good news for consumers.

Every food product label has a mandatory list of ingredients, detailing the contents of the pack, including preservatives and food colour. The label also includes a breakdown of nutritional values. Percentages of the protein, carbohydrate, fat and vitamin content are quantified, with portion sizes, or values, mentioned in grams. This makes it easier for you to understand the nutritional value per portion.

Another very important specification is the expiry date. It tells you how long that particular food item can be stored, so always make sure you check the expiry date. Some shops may keep stocks of soon-to-expire foodstuff in front and 'newer' supplies at the back, so be vigilant!

Once you pick up a product, look for 'how to stock' instructions on the label. For example, carton milk can be kept on the kitchen shelf till it is opened. When you cut open the carton, the milk has to be refrigerated. Even in the refrigerator, it has a limited shelf life and must be consumed within a given period.

Find the fine print

While you are on the COUNTDOWN, make the most of labels. Read the fine print, figure how best you can adapt the nutrition to your needs. While the calorie counts should get your attention, don't ignore details like sodium values. Packaged and preserved foods often have a high salt content, a factor that can lead to water retention and high blood pressure. Other red signals to look out for are high levels of saturated fats, trans-fats and cholesterol content.

If you are not sure about a particular product, just ask the store manager, or get in touch with the manufacturer. For instance, if you have food allergies, or are strictly vegetarian, you may have queries that need clarification. Many products have toll-free consumer care numbers printed on the label itself.

I have listed here some common nutritional values to look for.

Serving Size	1 cup
Servings per container	8 cups
Amount per serving	100 grams

Energy	1741 kJ
Protein	3.5 g
Carbohydrate –sugars	65.8 g 49.1
Fat –saturated fatty acid	15.2 g 3.6 g
Fibre	2.3 g
Sodium	0.1 g

Portion size and portions per container

Pay special attention to portion sizes, so that you are aware of the quantity you are consuming.

Energy

This line tells you the number of calories you are consuming for a given portion. The unit of measure is kilocalories, or kilojoules. 1 kcal = 4.2 kj

Fat

The fat component is measured per 100 g, or per portion. This can be broken into trans-fats, saturated and unsaturated fats. Opt for foods with higher levels of unsaturated fat, in the form of monounsaturates and polyunsaturates.

A high intake of saturated fats, commonly found in butter, cheese and meats, or trans-fat can raise low-density cholesterol levels and increase the risk for cardiovascular disease. Trans-fats are mostly found in fast-food items such as French fries, cakes, hamburgers and in packaged foods like crackers, chips, cookies and biscuits.

Sodium

This describes the salt content in the product. Keep in mind that sodium is a more concentrated form of salt.

1 gram sodium = 2.5 grams salt

Carbohydrates

Carbohydrates in the product could come from starches or from sugar. Some products will provide a breakdown of both sources.

Fibre

A fibre content of 3 g or above per portion is considered high-fibre food.

Protein

Your daily protein intake in grams should be approximately the same as your weight in kilograms.

SECTION III

FITNESS, A WAY OF LIFE

CHAPTER 16

WHY EXERCISE?

Your body is a complex, finely-tuned machine that can best be described as a living miracle! To a great degree, your health is determined by genetics. But it is important to know that lifestyle is an equally significant factor. While the scope of this book mainly covers diet, I feel exercise is a vital lifestyle component that has to be addressed. This is because diet alone, without exercise, cannot unlock the full potential of your weight loss goals. If your COUNTDOWN works in tandem with a sustained exercise programme, you will lose weight more rapidly and feel a lot fitter too!

To complement the COUNTDOWN, I have devised a comprehensive exercise routine to keep your body in peak condition. When your body gets wholesome food and the right amount of activity, you feel on top of the world. Your 'tune up' not only gives you physical benefits, but also improves your appearance. Okay, so you've heard all this before. Well, I have to tell you, there's more!

Did you know that exercise also works as a great mood-enhancer? When you exercise, blood flows to your brain and triggers the release of endorphins, which have the same effect on the mind as drugs prescribed for depression. Endorphins are hormones that produce a sense of well-being and reduce stress. Any physical activity—yoga, breathing techniques, stretching exercises, running or martial arts—can help you to de-stress and give you an exercise 'high'.

Look at tennis players or marathon runners. See how relaxed and confident they are—they walk tall, their eyes shine, their skin glows. Even their movements are harmonized, reflecting a better mind and body balance. They are experiencing the exercise high I am talking about. Once you start exercising regularly, you too will feel the same sense of exhilaration.

Why do so many exercisers drop out after a good start?

Many start a vigorous or complex training program, but fail to sustain the momentum. This could be due to injury, or mental and physical burn-out.

Take the case of Gautam. At 22, he was overweight and decided to exercise vigorously to lose weight. Every morning he would jog for 45 minutes and then, in the evening, he would run on the treadmill, at an incline, for another hour or so. Gautam dropped several kilos, but his knees and back started to hurt. He found it very hard to sustain his motivation levels and to continue pushing himself so much. So he stopped working out. The result? Not only did Gautam re-gain the weight he had lost, but he also lost faith in the efficacy of exercise.

I feel a fitness routine should be safe, effective and enjoyable. It should be a part of your lifestyle and fit seamlessly into your daily routine.

Mine is a case in point. From the age of 5, I trained for a rigorous swimming programme, to be a competitive swimmer in school. In addition, I played squash, badminton and table tennis. But because this activity was a regular part of my life, I never felt I was doing too much. For me, sports came naturally. All of us have varying threshold levels—some of us tend to be more physically inclined than others.

My childhood passion carried over into my adult years, as a career choice. Today, I enjoy nothing more than teaching and writing on wellness. I also cherish the hours I put in as a fitness instructor, guiding my students towards making better lifestyle choices.

My classes enable me to interact with over 200 students at any point in time. Students from all walks of life attend my classes in yoga, pilates, weights and aerobics. I also teach at a hospital and hold workshops for those with special needs such as arthritis, osteoporosis, back pain, high blood pressure, diabetes and other lifestyle-induced problems.

A little goes a long way

The debate is no longer 'to exercise or not to exercise' but how much, how often and with what intensity. The idea is to gain maximum benefit from a well-coordinated exercise regimen. I am now going to take you through some insights, based on real life cases, involving my students. (Names have been changed to maintain privacy.)

Sheila enrolled in my aerobics class with great enthusiasm. After a month or so, she asked me if the exercise was the reason she was gaining weight. I was surprised at her question and asked her to explain. Sheila had put on 1 kg in one month. I could see I had a very worried student on my hands!

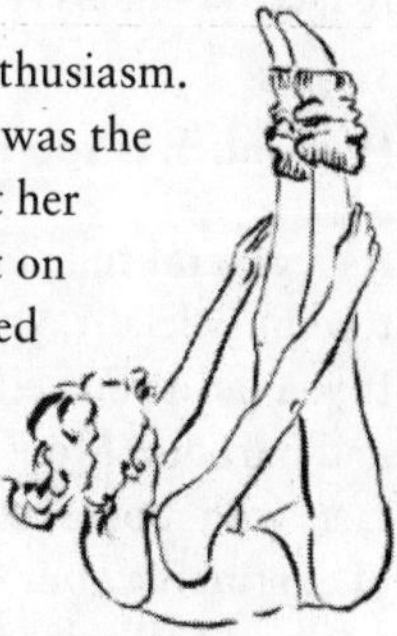

When I asked Sheila to give me an account of her daily food consumption, the penny dropped. She admitted to indulging in her favourite foods, because she assumed that exercise would burn off those extra calories. I had to remind her that, even with regular exercise, a high-calorie intake results in weight gain. So the moral of the story is: Don't go overboard just because you are exercising, always watch what you eat.

Another student, Suresh, went missing during the summer months. At first I thought he was away on vacation, then I bumped into him at a mall. He told me the 'killing heat' was the reason for his absence. He felt sick every time he exercised, more so because he spent a lot of time outdoors.

I gave Suresh a lecture in the middle of the mall, then and there! I agreed that exercising in hot weather can make you uncomfortable, but this was hardly an excuse to chuck up exercise.

I advised him to exercise indoors in an air-conditioned environment, or to start late evening walks instead. This way, his body was no longer exposed to high heat and humidity, which invariably leads to a rise in body temperature.

A few days later I saw Suresh again, running along a seaside promenade. He didn't see me—he was too busy jogging!

Another example: my student Cyrus is a real exercise junkie. He feels the more intense his workout, the more benefits he will gain. One day, he injured himself at the gym, and came to me for help. I advised him rest and recuperation. Then I suggested he should reduce the intensity of his workouts.

How much is too much?

As a general rule, moderate-intensity activity is best. If you exercise too superficially, you may not meet your fitness or weight-loss goals. If you push yourself too hard, you may increase your risk of injury and burnout. Moderate-intensity activity decreases these risks. In fact, with moderate-intensity exercise, you stand a better chance of continuing your exercise programme in the long run. When I explained all this to Cyrus, it made sense to him and he toned down the intensity of his exercise regimen.

You too can follow these guidelines to give yourself a moderate-intensity workout.

- Feel muscles work, but not to the point of agonizing pain.

- Use the 'talk test', which means you can carry on a brief conversation in short sentences, but cannot sing a song.
- Design your fitness routine around your individual health status and fitness goals.

Make an appointment—with yourself!

Schedule 'workout' in your daily planner. Make exercise an important part of your daily life and write it down so that you are more likely to keep the 'appointment'.

If you are a morning person, schedule your workouts early in the day, so that you kick-start your day with exercise. If you like to end the day on a high note, plan to exercise in the evening. If you prefer to break away at noon, do so. Basically, find a time slot that suits you, then stay with it.

Don't be a sitting target

If you sit around doing nothing, you become an easy target. A sedentary lifestyle attracts all kinds of health problems, like obesity, osteoporosis, diabetes, hypercholesterolemia and high blood pressure. Other common problems that inactive people suffer from include mood swings, lethargy, depression, aches and pains. You get the general idea—so get moving!

- Exercise promotes weight loss
- Exercise reduces the risk of heart disease, diabetes, high blood pressure and osteoporosis
- Exercise decreases bad (LDL) cholesterol and increases good (HDL) cholesterol
- Exercise corrects posture
- Exercise improves stamina
- Exercise boosts immunity

Make the right moves

Increase your activity levels whenever possible. Every little bit counts, because whenever you move, you are using energy and burning off calories. Walking, active chores at home, gardening, spring cleaning the house, climbing the stairs, walking your dog, carrying your shopping home, dancing—they all count as exercise.

Cooking	148 calories per hour
Cleaning the home	207 calories per hour
Childcare—dressing/feeding, while standing	207 calories per hour
Dancing	266 calories per hour

Fit tips

- If you are sitting, get up and walk around the room every one hour. Remember to do this when you are watching television or at the office. This helps to keep your blood circulation going.
- Take the stairs, rather than the elevator. With practice you will be able to do this without getting out of breath.
- Chores like gardening or walking the dog are a great way to keep fit.
- Remember to keep your abs tucked in at all times. This will help strengthen the abs muscles.

Apple versus pear

Are you apple-shaped or pear-shaped? If your shoulders are more developed than your hips, you are a classic 'apple'. If your hips are heavier, it makes you a 'pear'. The pattern of fat distribution can actually define your health risk for certain diseases. Excess abdominal fat, or an apple-shaped body, known as the android type of obesity, is associated with an increased risk of heart disease.

In contrast, if you gain weight on the hips and thighs, resembling a pear, known as the gynoid type of obesity, you do not run the same risk of heart ailments. Usually, due to genetic factors, men are prone to storing fat in the abdominal region and women on the hips and thighs.

How many inches did you measure?

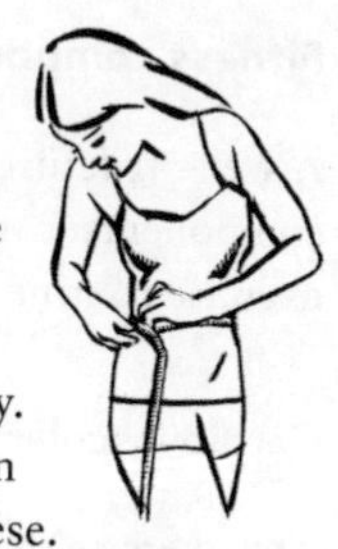

Take a measuring tape around the circumference of your waist. Pull the tape maintaining an appropriate tension and note the measurement.

This is one of the key measures used to assess obesity. A waist circumference of more than 40 inches in men and more than 35 inches in women is considered obese.

Body fat percentage

What is your body fat percentage? If you are able to get your body fat percentage analysed using special equipment, take a look at this chart for a better understanding of what the percentages indicate.

Women

Essential fat: 10–13 per cent
Athletes: 14–20 per cent
Fit people: 21–24 per cent
Average: 25–31 per cent
Obese: 32 per cent and higher

Men

Essential fat: 2–5 per cent
Athletes: 6–13 per cent
Fit people: 14–17 per cent
Average: 18–24 per cent
Obese: 25 per cent and higher

Aim to improve your body composition by lowering your fat percentage and increasing your percentage of muscle mass.

Fitness components

A well-structured exercise plan should include 3 main fitness components: cardiovascular fitness, strength training and an exercise routine for flexibility.

Cardiovascular Fitness

Any exercise that conditions the heart is called aerobic or cardiovascular exercise. Examples are walking, jogging, cycling, swimming or skipping. The heart is the most active muscle in the body and regular exercise helps your heart to function more efficiently. To keep your heart healthy, you need to exercise for a minimum of 30 minutes every day, 7 days of the week. This maintains the heart, lungs and circulatory system in great condition.

Strength Training

Strength training enhances muscle strength, increases bone density and helps to keep the joints in peak condition. Other benefits include a boost for your metabolism, improved posture and a more sculpted body. You can strength train on various types of equipment in a health club, gym or at home. (Please note a home workout routine is given in the Home Gym Exercise chapter.)

After you strength train, it is important to rest your muscles. Working out on alternate days provides time for recuperation and repair of muscle tissue. It is therefore ideal to train every major muscle group 2 to 3 times per week, but no more.

Flexibility Exercises

Often neglected, flexibility is an aspect of fitness that is as important as cardiovascular and strength training.

A flexible body is supple and free from muscular stress. Yoga uses stretching in a highly scientific form, to achieve benefits such as increased blood flow and nutrient supply to joint structures, relaxing the muscles, mobilizing the joints and improving posture.

Exercise helps create a calorie deficit

To lose weight you need to create a calorie deficit. A weight loss of 1 to 2 pounds per week is ideal. To lose 1 pound a week, you need to cut 500 calories a day. That makes a total of 3500 calories a week. The best way to achieve this is by reducing your calorie intake and increasing calorie expenditure through exercise.

If you cut 250 calories with reduced food consumption, and burn 250 calories with daily exercise, you will create a calorie deficit of 500 calories per day. Do this every day and you have a 3500 calorie deficit, which works out to 1 pound in 1 week.

On your COUNTDOWN diet, you are creating a calorie deficit between 300 to 700 calories per day. Exercise burns up another 250–300 calories per day, giving you a total deficit of 500 to 1000 calories in a day.

3500 calories	= 1 pound weight
1000 calories @ 7 days	= 7000 calories or 2 pounds weight

In 7 days, that is one week, you therefore lose 2 pounds, which is approximately 1 kilo. As you can see, exercise plays a crucial role in weight loss. It is factored into the entire COUNTDOWN diet plan, to enable you to get the weight loss results you want. If you retain this weight loss rate throughout the FOUR-WEEK COUNTDOWN, it adds up to a total weight loss of about 4 kilos in one month.

Guaranteed weight loss with exercise

Include a moderate-intensity cardiovascular exercise routine, for example, a brisk walk for one hour, 7 days a week. You can split your workout routine into two 30-minute sessions or even into three 20-minute sessions.

In addition, do a strength routine twice, or three times a week, for 20 to 30 minutes. Include stretching exercises at the end of your workout, or better still, do a yoga routine two to three times a week, to keep the body supple.

Always start your workout with a warm-up. 5 minutes of spot marching is an ideal warm-up and you could end with a 5-minute cool-down, where you use the last 5 minutes of your exercise to gradually taper off the intensity of the workout.

MAKE YOUR WORKOUT WORK FOR YOU

Suggested 7-day Workout Plan

Monday: Walk 1 hour +
Strength Workout 30 minutes

Tuesday: Walk 1 hour +
Yoga or Stretch 30 minutes

Wednesday: Walk 1 hour +
Strength Workout 30 minutes

Thursday: Walk 1 hour

Friday: Walk 1 hour +
Yoga or Stretch 30 minutes

Saturday: Walk 1 hour

Sunday: Walk 1 hour +
Yoga or Stretch 30 minutes

A word of caution

When starting out, begin at a level you are comfortable with. Then, once you determine your fitness level, progress gradually. It's smart to get specific guidelines from your family physician about how much you can do, based on age, your aptitude, and your recent medical history.

Progressing too soon and doing too much: is it a good thing?

While you may set ambitious goals for yourself, remember, your body may not be able to keep up! Doing too much too fast can deplete the body of its energy reserves and lead to fatigue. Then as immunity levels go down, your body succumbs more easily to infection and illness.

Aim for a burn rate of 250–300 calories a day. The calorie-burning activities listed here will help you figure how much to do. Remember, however, that calories burned are also determined by factors such as body weight, fitness level and intensity of exercise.

Walk: Just put on your walking shoes and walk anywhere, anytime.
Calories burnt: 300 an hour

Uphill Walk: This increases walking intensity and shapes the legs and hips.
Calories burnt: 400 an hour

Swim: Challenge your muscles in water.
A safe, low-impact exercise that works the whole body.
Calories burnt: 400 an hour.

Cycle: Indoor or outdoor cycling is a great exercise for toning the lower body.
Calories burnt: 350 an hour

Tennis/Squash/Badminton: Nothing beats the thrill of sport.
Calories burnt: 400 an hour

Skip/Speed Jog (interval): Burn more calories in 25 minutes by interval training.
Skip for 2 minutes. Jog (fast jog) for 3 minutes. Repeat for 25 minutes.
Calories burnt: 300 in 25 minutes

Jog on a trampoline: Bounce on a trampoline.
Calories burnt: 300 an hour

Run: Pick up pace, feel the power in movement. A great exercise high!
Calories burnt: 400 an hour.

Punch & Kick: Buy a punching bag and gloves, then punch and kick in turn.
Calories burnt: 450 an hour

MYTH BUSTER

Get rid of that belly fat in a jiffy! Lose those extra inches in one week! How I lost 90 pounds in 90 days! No, this is not me talking. These are some sample headlines you will find if you Google 'weight loss'. Every promo makes it sound like weight loss is the easiest thing to achieve. If it were so, there would be no fat people on planet earth, right?

But you and I know better. You know, as you go through my FOUR-WEEK COUNTDOWN, that you have to slog it out, sweat it out, for every kilo you lose. Weight loss is no picnic!

But the media hypes up the myth so successfully, you end up believing it. Other times, some dieticians, trainers and fitness experts perpetuate certain myths, because it is in their interest to do so.

For example, dieticians often advise against strength training, as it makes you 'put on weight'. What they may not tell you is that the weight you gain is healthy muscle mass, not fat. A good dietician-supervised weight loss plan should include balanced meals and strength training, so that you do not lose muscle or weaken your bones, just because you happen to be on a diet.

Over the years, my students have come to me with queries that I have answered one-on-one. This chapter now gives me the opportunity to address several such questions, frequently asked, and debunk some myths once and for all. What I have tried to do here is clarify misconceptions, or amplify certain points that are difficult to grasp, to help you understand how exercise works.

Q. I have recently signed up for an exercise class but I find exercise increases my appetite and makes me hungry. I am eating more and have put on weight instead of knocking it off. So why should I bother to exercise?

A. Initially, when you start exercising, you may feel hungrier. This is because your body's metabolic rate increases with exercise. But over time, as you become physically fit, your body will adapt to the increased physical activity and your appetite will stabilize.

Exercise doesn't give you a licence to indulge. If you indulge, you are bound to gain weight.

FACT FILE

Research shows that sticking to an exercise plan is the strongest predictor of long-term success in weight management.

Q. I lose weight much faster when I go on a crash diet, but exercising just doesn't do it for me . . .

A. Exercise not only shapes the body but also helps decrease levels of body fat. Drastic dieting, on the other hand, also drastically lowers the metabolic rate and thereby slows down the fat burning process.

FACT FILE

In non-exercising dieters, about 25 per cent of weight lost will be due to loss of muscle mass. But in people who exercise and diet, only about 8 per cent of weight lost will be due to loss of muscle mass. Exercise prevents loss of muscle mass—a very important factor in staying healthy.

Why is muscle mass so important? Because muscle mass helps burn calories. Also, more muscle means a faster metabolism. This is precisely the reason why your metabolic rate can increase by 25 per cent after exercise, as muscle requires more oxygen and calories to maintain itself, while fat requires very little.

One of my students, Rani, trained with me for over a year. I can vouch for the fact that she worked out consistently, and as a result, lost several inches. But it didn't show on her scale! Rani was not complaining, but she was curious to know how it was possible to fit into the slimmest of jeans, and yet not have lost weight.

I explained it to her. Her weight had not altered, but her body composition had. Her consistent exercise routine had shaped up her muscles, strengthened her bones, and melted away the subcutaneous fat under the skin. So what she saw in the mirror was a toned and slender body, even though her weight had remained constant.

The body is composed of fat and fat-free mass, such as bones, tendons and muscles. When you exercise, the fat decreases substantially and the fat-free mass increases. To lose weight on the scale, you must exercise, and simultaneously make an effort to cut back on caloric intake, through a diet plan.

Q. One question that is repeated with alarming regularity is the 'muscle to fat' story. So many students come up to me with this: 'When I stop weight training, will my muscle turn into fat?'

A. Simply put, no. Muscle and fat have separate properties. Muscle cannot turn into fat and fat cannot be converted into muscle. When you stop exercising, the trained muscle eventually gets back to its pre-exercise level.

Q. I need to lose 7 kilos. I really enjoy exercising, especially after spending long hours in the office; exercise is a great stress buster for me. But I just can't seem to control my food portions and at meal times, I forget all about dieting. I am prepared to exercise even more, as long as I can lose weight, but please don't ask me to diet!

A. Exercise alone is NOT enough to lose weight. Exercise will help you get into shape, burn fat, even improve your body composition. But to lose weight, there's no getting away from the fact that you need to watch your diet as well.

Keep in mind, once you've decided to lose weight, nothing and nobody can stop you! Constantly remind yourself of all the benefits of weight loss. Think how great you are going to look and feel . . . a positive spirit is the most potent ingredient for weight loss.

Fit Tip

Consult a trainer. It is a good idea to consult a qualified fitness professional to meet your goals. Sometimes, you need to be sure that your workouts are working for you.

70 per cent Diet + 30 per cent Exercise = Weight loss

CHAPTER 17

WHAT A RELIEF!

Special treatment for special needs

Many of you may assume that if you have any sort of health problem, or physical disability, you are not a candidate for exercise. Wrong! You can plan an exercise routine to specifically target your areas of concern. In fact, exercise can even control the symptoms to a great extent and, in some cases, correct the problem altogether.

Conditions such as high blood pressure, diabetes, backache, arthritis, hypertension or high cholesterol can be very effectively treated with exercise. In my experience as a clinical exercise specialist, I have seen the most amazing results in clients who take up some form of physical activity to counter their health problems. This particularly applies to lifestyle-related diseases, where it is just a matter of knowing which exercise to focus on, and what to avoid.

I hate to bring this up, but some people tend to imagine aches and pains that do not exist. This means you are basically looking for an excuse to skip exercise. When you do this, you are only cheating yourself. Exercise as a form of therapy is a natural, proven method of staying fit, so why deprive yourself of it?

Sometimes, circumstances play a role in curtailing your physical activity. Take the case of my school friend, Radha. She was a keen sportsperson in her growing years. In fact, as kids, we both played squash in school. Over time, I lost touch with her. I heard she had had a knee injury and had stopped playing completely.

When I met Radha last year, I was shocked to see her condition—she had gained an enormous amount of weight and looked peaky and haggard. She had given up her squash game and was getting no other form of exercise.

I strongly recommended that she get back into some sort of exercise programme. Squash was no longer an option, but there were other alternatives she could try. For starters, I suggested walking, swimming or cycling. I also advised her to begin a strength training routine with a qualified trainer. Leg-strengthening exercises would strengthen her leg muscles and offer support to her knee joints. Upper body and abdominal exercises would take care of overall fitness.

Thankfully, Radha followed my advice. Today, she is in great shape. We met recently at a school reunion, and I have to tell you, she was the toast of the evening!

Like Radha, there are many who, despite their health condition, will benefit from exercise. Always remember to consult your physician before you start on any exercise plan, because it is very important to factor your health history and current medical condition into the routine.

Arthritis

Arthritis is characterized by inflammation, pain or tenderness that causes stiffness in the body joints. Commonly affected parts are the major weight-bearing joints, such as the hips, knees, spine and shoulder.

If you are an arthritis sufferer, the worst mistake you can make is to get into a vicious cycle of inactivity. The more you avoid exercise, the weaker your body will get. In time, your sedentary lifestyle will lead to increased stiffness, reduced strength and compromised cardiovascular fitness. It's a downward spiral from there because, with neglect, your arthritis condition can only get from bad to worse.

I am an arthritis sufferer. What do I do?

Loosen up with daily stretching

The most important exercises are stretching exercises which preserve a range of motion and flexibility around each joint. Even inflamed joints can be put through a gentle stretching routine with the assistance of a therapist.

Gentle strength training helps

Strength training exercises using light weights is an excellent way to build bone strength. Do these exercises only when pain and joint inflammation are under control, and in consultation with your physician.

Low-impact cardiovascular exercise

In the past, aerobic exercise was excluded for arthritis suffers, for fear of aggravating joint pain. Now, however, aerobic exercise is considered safe and effective, particularly when joint inflammation is not acute. Low-impact cardiovascular exercises such as swimming, cycling and walking are also wonderful ways to exercise your joints and improve fitness.

> Swimming is a non-weight bearing activity that places the minimum stress on your joints. Working out in water is therefore a great exercise option for anyone with sports injuries, back or joint problems.

Stress-free arthritis management

- If you are overweight, you are further straining your joints. When you reduce some weight, the pressure on the joints is also automatically reduced, giving them some relief.
- Get the right kind of footwear. Well-fitting shoes with good support eases the pain and helps to keep your feet in good condition.
- Warm baths, ice packs or heat pads can help soothe joint pain.
- Learn to listen to your body signals. If you over-burden your joints with continuous, stressful movement, the pain will tell you to slow down.

Osteoporosis

Osteoporosis is a bone-weakening disease that develops gradually, making the bones fragile and susceptible to fractures. Women are more prone to develop this condition, especially after age 30, when they begin to lose bone density.

Weight bearing exercises, such as light resistance training, can increase calcium deposits in the bones. Even something as simple as walking, which is a weight bearing exercise, will help strengthen your bones.

The popular perception is that weight bearing exercises are only for the fit but the truth is, anyone, at any age, can practise a light resistance training routine.

FACT FILE

1 in 3 women and 1 in 12 men over the age of 50 develop fragile bones. This makes them more susceptible to osteoporosis.

Food for the bones

Calcium

Inadequate calcium intake can contribute to brittle bones. Research shows that many women consume less than half the amount of calcium required to maintain healthy bones. Depending on your age, an appropriate calcium intake falls between 1000 and 1200 mg per day.

> Milk, yoghurt, orange juice, cheese, sardine, oyster, green vegetables, beans and broccoli are some calcium-rich foods.

Vitamin D

Vitamin D is needed to absorb calcium. The early morning rays of the sun are gentle, yet provide the valuable vitamin D needed for healthy bones. Do not, however, expose yourself to the sun for long periods. The recommended daily intake of vitamin D is 1000 ug.

> Milk, egg yolk, tuna and salmon contain vitamin D.

Diabetes

If you are diabetic, you are already aware of the dangers associated with the condition. You have to take extra care to guard yourself against problems like kidney failure, nerve disorders, eye problems and heart disease. Exercise helps to improve glucose regulation, reduces the risk for heart disease, hypertension, cholesterol levels and excess weight.

The exercise timings, the amount of insulin injected and the injection site are important factors to be considered before exercise.

- Exercise regularly and lead an active lifestyle
- Plan healthy meals and follow regular meal timings
- Take medication as prescribed by your doctor

FACT FILE

In the US, a study conducted by the Diabetes Prevention Program (DPP) found that a modest weight loss of 5 per cent to 7 per cent of your body weight, achieved with diet and exercise, can delay and possibly prevent type 2 diabetes.

What is the duration, frequency and type of exercise you, as a diabetic, can safely do? 30 to 60 minutes of moderate-paced intensity exercises 5 to 7 days a week is recommended. If you are not accustomed to physical activity, you may start with a shorter duration and work your way up.

Hypertension

High blood pressure overstrains the heart, increasing the risk of heart disease and stroke. The good news is, exercise can actually lower high blood pressure. Regular, low-impact aerobic activity can reduce both systolic and diastolic blood pressure by an average of 10mm Hg.

Endurance activities such as walking, cycling and swimming, or low intensity aerobic exercises, like working out on a treadmill, are recommended. You may also do weight training exercises using light resistance. Heavy resistance weight training exercises are NOT recommended as these can elevate blood pressure.

Frequency 30–60 minutes 4 to 6 days a week
Always include a gradual 10-minute warm-up before getting started.

High cholesterol

The cholesterol level in your body is determined partly by genetics and partly by lifestyle factors. Diet, exercise and even psychological stress can contribute to a high cholesterol build-up. You may not be aware that you have a cholesterol problem, as it can occur gradually, without any symptoms showing.

An annual test with your physician is the only way to determine your cholesterol level. This is a must, to make sure you are in the clear. If you do have a problem, it is even more important to know, so that you can take the necessary precautions to control the condition.

What is the best way to lower blood cholesterol?

For those of you who are overweight, dietary reduction of saturated fat, exercise and weight loss has to be the primary goal.

Current guidelines recommend that total cholesterol in the body should not exceed 200 mg per deciliter (mg/dl). If your 'total cholesterol level' is between 200 to 239 mg/dl, you are at an 'increased risk' for developing coronary heart disease. If your 'total cholesterol level' is 240 mg/dl or above, you are in the 'high risk' category.

Exercise greatly helps in lowering cholesterol levels. Regular exercise, such as brisk walking, jogging, cycling or swimming, cuts the risk of hypercholesterolemia.

Frequency 30–60 minutes 7 days a week

FACT FILE

Weight loss, especially **fat loss around the waist and abdomen**, is associated with an increase in HDL cholesterol, the good cholesterol. It also signifies a reduction in LDL cholesterol, the bad cholesterol, and triglyceride levels.

CHAPTER 18

HOME GYM EXERCISE ROUTINE

Are you like most people, who include a walk and yoga into your fitness plan, but skip the strength training? If that is the case, it's time to revamp your routine! You must incorporate a strength training routine to keep fit. Once you start including strength training exercises into your workout, you are less likely to suffer from bone injuries or fractures. Conditions such as osteoporosis and back pain can also be prevented or reduced with regular strength training exercises.

You might not like working out at a gym for various reasons—distance, convenience, the time factor, overloud music, overcrowded workout floors, and so on. But that does not have to stop you from achieving your fitness goals. The fact is, you can get into great shape without ever stepping foot into a gym.

So lose no time—get ready to lose the kilos instead!

I have put together a simple exercise schedule that is easy and fun. The 13 exercises that follow are designed to work all your major muscle groups. It is therefore important to build each one into your regular routine, so as not to neglect any part of the body.

STRENGTH TRAINING WORKOUT

Warm-up: Start with a 5-minute warm-up by walking/marching briskly.
Frequency: 3 times a week, on alternate days.

1. Schedule your workout
Treat your home workout like a regular appointment. Pencil in your workout in your daily planner, otherwise you'll always find excuses to dodge your exercise session.

2. Tell your family this is your time off
This is not the time to help around household chores. Make it a rule—this is your time and space to look and feel good.

3. Switch on music that you enjoy
Music makes workouts more enjoyable and you don't realize how time slips by.

Home props

- Dumbbells or 2 water bottles (500 ml each)
- A mat or carpet
- A step or chair

Strength Workout Exercises

1. PUSH-UPS repeat 16 counts

A wonderful exercise that shapes the upper body!

BENEFIT: Strengthens the chest, shoulder and arms

Place your hands on the floor under your shoulders (keeping them wider than shoulder-width apart) and keep your back straight. Bend your elbows as you bring your chest closer towards the floor and then return to starting position.

2. BENT OVER LATERAL repeat 16 counts

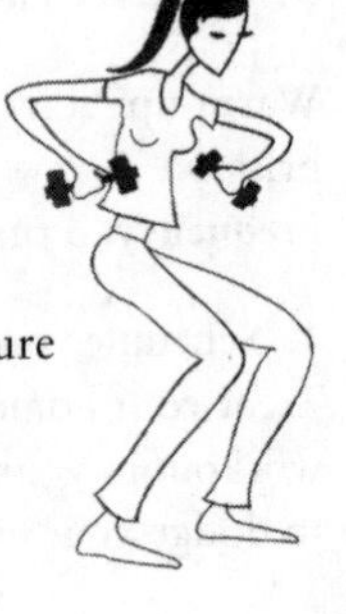

To get the most from this exercise, concentrate on working your back muscles. This exercise helps improves posture.

BENEFIT: Strengthens back muscles, improves posture

Stand tall, holding weights in both hands. Lean forward slightly from the hips, keep back straight. Bend the elbows and lift your arms laterally, pull weights up till your waist. Gently lower hands.

3. BICEP CURL repeat 16 counts

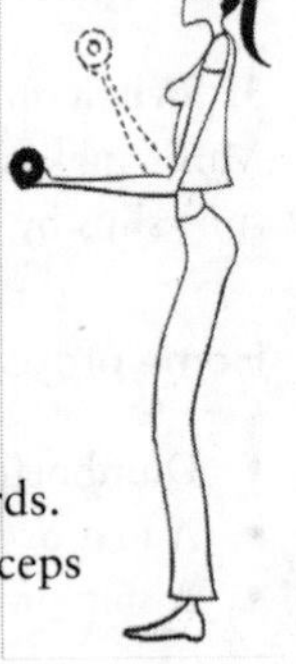

This is a great exercise for creating definition and strength in the biceps. You can actually see the muscle definition when you concentrate on tensing the biceps.

BENEFIT: Tones and shapes front arm muscles

Hold weights in both hands, with palms turned outwards. Bend the elbows towards your shoulders, tensing the biceps as you lift upwards and then lower.

4. TRICEP DIPS repeat 16 counts

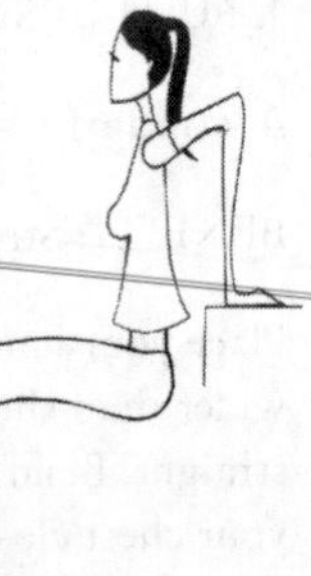

This upper arm exercise works the back of the arms. These muscles need to be strengthened as they are usually not as strong as the front of the arm.

BENEFIT: Tones the triceps

Sit on the edge of a chair or step and grip the edge with your hands. Bend your elbows as you lower your hips towards the floor. Use your triceps to push back up to starting position.

5. SHOULDER PRESS repeat 16 counts

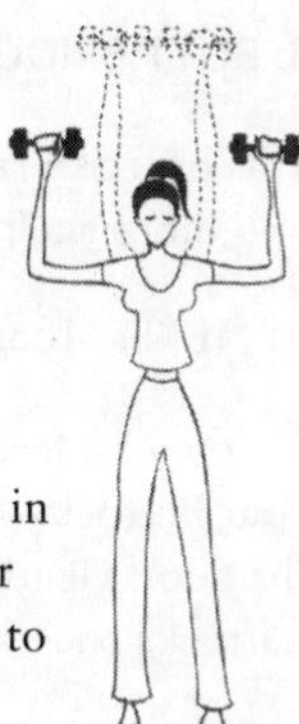

Toned shoulders help create a sculpted appearance—the waist appears narrower and the body looks more streamlined.

BENEFIT: Strengthens shoulders

Stand tall. Hold weights in both hands, palms facing in front, elbows bent just below shoulder level. Lift your arms slowly above your head. Then lower arms back to shoulder level.

6. CALF RAISE repeat 16 counts

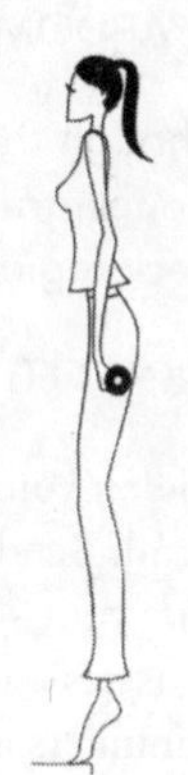

Persevere with this exercise, because this is one of the quickest and most effective ways to tone the calves. In a month, you will see the difference.

BENEFIT: Shapes and strengthens calf muscles

Stand tall, with shoulders back and chest lifted. Stand on a step. Come up on your toes and, balancing on the balls of your feet, lift your heels as high as possible. Slowly lower your heels.

7. POWER LUNGES repeat 16 counts

This is an excellent exercise to shape the thighs and hips.

BENEFIT: Strengthens and tones the hips and thighs

Hold weights in your hands, keeping feet shoulder-width apart. Bring one food forward into a lunge position, both your knees are bent forming a 90-degree angle. Return to starting position and switch legs.

8. BUTT BRIDGE repeat 16 counts

This exercise targets the muscles of the hips, giving them a firmer and more sculpted appearance.

BENEFIT: Tones and strengthens buttocks and back of the thighs

Lie on mat, feet shoulder-width apart. Contract your buttocks and slowly lift them off the floor. Gently lower your buttocks back onto mat.

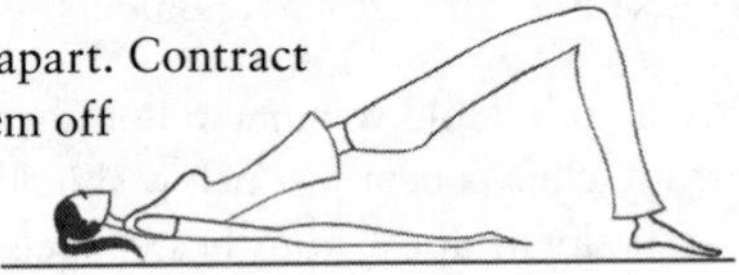

9. ABDOMINAL CRUNCH repeat 16 counts

Though this is a basic abdominal exercise, it is very effective. Concentrate on good form, and be careful to avoid stress to the neck region, especially as you lift your shoulders off the floor.

BENEFIT: Tones and tightens abdominal muscles

Lie on your back with your hands placed behind your head. Bend knees, with feet shoulder-width apart. Lift your shoulders slowly, feel your abdominal muscles contract. Slowly lower shoulders down. Breathe out as you lift, breathe in as you lower.

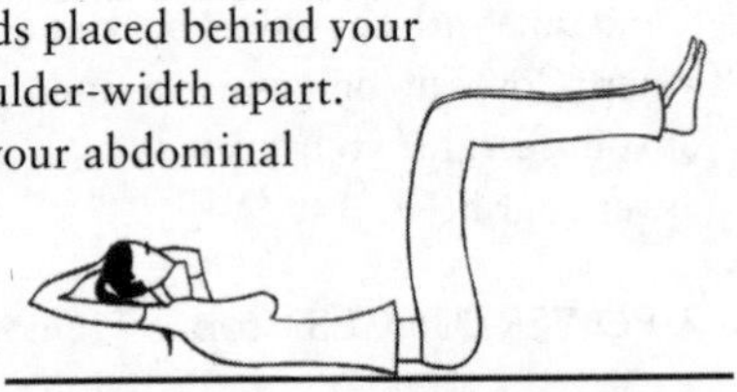

Training Tip: As you come up, use the hands only to support your head and not to tilt your chin towards your chest. You can also increase the challenge by raising the legs and bending the knees to a 90-degree angle.

10. REVERSE CURL repeat 16 counts

A great exercise addition to the basic crunch. The reverse curl places no stress on the neck or shoulders as they are resting on the mat. This exercise targets the same abdominal muscle as the abs crunch, but here you initiate the movement from the lower part of the abs.

BENEFIT: Tones and shapes abs

Lie on your back with your hands by your side, palms facing down. Gently lift your legs off the floor, with knees slightly bent. Tilt your pelvis and slowly bring your legs towards you and return back to starting position.

11. OBLIQUE CRUNCH repeat 16 counts

Aim to get the shoulder as close as possible to your knee. The closer you get, the better it is for your waist.

BENEFIT: Works the waist muscles

Lie on your back, with knees bent and feet shoulder-width apart. Place your arms behind your head, raise your shoulders and twist, bringing the left shoulder towards the right knee. Then twist to the other side, bringing the right shoulder to the left knee.

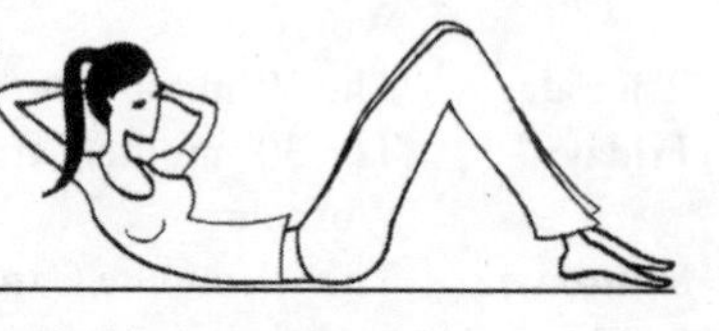

12. BACK EXTENSION repeat 16 counts

This exercise concentrates on strengthening your back, improving posture and body alignment. While doing this movement keep your eyes focused on the mat.

BENEFIT: Strengthens back muscles

Lie on your stomach. Keep elbows bent, with forearms on the mat. Slowly lift the shoulders and chest off the floor and then lower them.

Training Tip: Keep the head, neck and spine aligned while lifting. Do not strain the neck muscles by lifting and tilting the neck backwards

The 30-minute Indoor Cardio Workout

March walk: 10 minutes
Jog in place: 5 minutes
Knee lifts: 5 minutes
Brisk march in place: 10 minutes

Suggested 7-day Indoor Workout Plan

Monday:	The 30-minute Cardio Workout + Home Strength Workout
Tuesday:	The 30-minute Cardio Workout
Wednesday:	The 30-minute Cardio Workout + Home Strength Workout
Thursday:	The 30-minute Cardio Workout
Friday:	The 30-minute Cardio Workout + Home Strength Workout
Saturday:	The 30-minute Cardio Workout
Sunday:	Stretch and relax

CHAPTER 19

SPA-SCOPE

When it comes to de-stressing in a modern world, spas offer the latest in health and wellness treatments. But in case you were not aware, the spa has actually been around for thousands of years! The spa celebrates its origins in water. 'Espa' is the Latin word for fountain. Sanus Per Aquam—SPA—means health through water. From Roman baths to the mineral springs of Switzerland, from Turkish hamams to the communal hot spring baths of Japan, hydrotherapy is an ancient wellness concept our ancestors have enjoyed through the centuries.

The spa as we know it today is like a holistic healing centre. It's the place for rest and rejuvenation, the getaway that offers a respite from the demands of daily life. Once you enroll in a spa, the idea is to unwind in sylvan surroundings, let go of life's problems, and get yourself pampered from head to toe!

In India, the spa culture is highly evolved. If you suffer from aches and pains, massage therapy is available. If you want to lose weight, 'diet' spas help you to shed the kilos. Even specialized therapies—curing skin problems like acne, treating disorders like arthritis and rheumatism, or offering a full detox regimen—can be part of a spa package.

If chronic pain is your problem, with headaches, neck, shoulder or back pain, chances are the pain originates from tense or contracted muscles. Releasing the tension from these muscles is an integral part of massage therapy.

Did you know that massage can be done in a hundred different ways?

By definition, massage is the intentional and systematic manipulation of the soft tissues of the body, to enhance health and healing. It is a form of therapy which uses different techniques to promote increased blood flow and subsequent healing.

The uniqueness of this therapy is that it doesn't just affect the skin—the largest organ in our body—but the entire system gets an overhaul. You could benefit from a weekly massage regimen, or fortnightly sessions, to help you relax and re-charge.

To help you make a choice, I am covering some popular types of massage here.

Deep-tissue massage

A slow, focused style of massage that often works across the direction of the muscle fibres to release chronic muscle tension and break up calcified bruises in the muscles.

Sports massage

A specialized form of Swedish massage developed for athletes, but useful for anyone with chronic pain, stiffness or injury. The massage is usually localized or focused on the problem area. Sports massage is also useful before and after sporting events, in which case the areas addressed are those that are used in the particular activity.

Lymphatic massage

Gentle, rhythmic, repetitive strokes stimulate and promote the movement of lymphatic fluids, the body's filtration and infection control system. This is especially useful for those who suffer from edema (excess fluid and swelling).

Swedish massage

This type of massage employs a combination of long strokes and kneading, generally in the direction of the heart. It uses oil as a lubricant. The emphasis is on increasing circulation and relaxing the nervous system.

Underwater massage

Water treatments can be used to alleviate a variety of health problems. A form of underwater massage is the 'hydrotherapy bath', consisting of several water jets. The pressure of the water from these water jets promotes circulation, provides relaxation and results in elimination of toxins and reduction of cellulite.

Shiatsu

Shiatsu is a Japanese word meaning 'finger pressure'. The application of pressure is the underlying principle of Shiatsu. The treatment, approach and philosophy are similar to acupuncture, with the use of energy channels and pressure points, but the pressure applied is with the fingers instead of needles. In addition to application of pressure, assisted stretches are given, to help relieve body stiffness.

Thai massage

A fluid style of massage developed 2500 years ago in Buddhist monasteries, as a form of healing practice. This type of massage uses pressure points to actively stretch muscles and ligaments.

Through manipulation of muscles, the spine is elongated, and the entire body is stretched to relieve tension.

Ayurvedic massage

Ayurvedic massage, developed 5000 years ago, offers physical and mental benefits. The purpose of the massage is to assist the body and its organs to repair and renew themselves. Practitioners concentrate on energy centres and muscle manipulation, to treat individual needs. During this process, warm herbal oil is lavishly applied on the body to assist in the therapeutic cure.

Dhara, nasyam, pizhichil, navarakizi, lepam, udvardanam, body scrubs, body wraps are some of the treatments your ayurvedic doctor may recommend.

Reflexology

Reflexology taps into the body's reflex network, stimulating the pressure sensors located on the soles of the feet. Every pressure point in the foot connects to a particular part of the body, with demarcated 'zones' for the internal organs as well.

Pressure is applied to the feet using specific thumb, finger and hand techniques. Using just the right amount of pressure is essential, as too much pressure can lead to injury. Gentle manipulation of joints also provides relaxation and relief to the foot. Oils, creams and lotions are generally avoided in traditional reflexology work.

You should always inform your reflexologist if you feel any unusual pain when pressure is applied. Each session generally takes 30 minutes to one hour.

FACT FILE

Traditional Chinese medicine has gained a huge following in the West. In Chinese medicine, charts dating back thousands of years target certain points in the body called 'trigger points' for energy channels. This is based on the knowledge that these points correspond to internal organs and joints, and that manipulating them can have direct benefits on the corresponding body parts.

CHAPTER 20

SAUNAS & STEAM BATHS

Saunas and steam baths can also be called sweat baths because both stimulate the sweat glands to produce heavy perspiration. Age-old traditions in sauna and steam are used to relax and detoxify the body and enable better blood circulation.

Do saunas and steam baths 'melt away fat'?

No. Health professionals have extensively investigated the use of saunas and steam baths in the context of weight loss. What emerges is that yes, you will weigh slightly less when your sauna session is over. This is because when you are in a sauna, there is a high volume of continuous water loss from the body, in the form of perspiration.

The loss is temporary however, for as soon as you eat or drink anything, the fluids in the body are replaced, and body weight reverts to pre-sauna levels.

What is the difference between steam and sauna?

The sauna uses dry heat and is referred to as a dry hot-air bath. In this system, air is heated in a cubicle for a specific length of time, allowing the sauna occupant to keep sweating continuously for that given period. For some, particularly for those with respiratory problems, this can become claustrophobic and uncomfortable.

In a steam bath, the heat is moist. The steam bath uses a steam generator to produce a continuous supply of steam. While the sauna has very low humidity, the steam bath has high humidity. In a steam bath, the steam builds up to create a humidity level of around 100 per cent. The difference in temperatures is also significant. A steam bath, because of the moisture, retains heat at 40 degrees centigrade or so. But the dry heat of a sauna can boost temperatures to up to 60 degrees centigrade.

CHAPTER 21

GIZMOS & GADGETS

A quick lowdown on equipment like vibration machines, sauna belts, massagers and the like. Gizmos and gadgets promise to work off those kilos from your body, with no effort on your part, but how effective are they? What's the fine print on these devices?

Can massage chairs and vibration belts actually guarantee sustainable weight loss?

The answer is NO. There is a very good reason why diet books sell more than vibration belts and massage chairs! Diet and exercise are the only proven way to lose weight and sustain the weight loss. You have to put in effort to see results. I'm sorry, but that is just how the cookie crumbles and the sooner you accept it, the better!

How far do machines act as a substitute to exercise?

Sauna belts, vibration machines and walkers can stimulate blood circulation and induce sweating. When you sweat, you shed your water weight, and this may give an illusion of weight loss. But these machines can NEVER be a substitute for exercise. Regular activity, in the form of cardio workouts, stretching exercises or yoga, is what you need to burn fat and shape up.

Why are these products so heavily marketed and advertised? Do they not live up to the hype?

If a headline reads, 'Lose 10 pounds in 2 weeks' or a television show promises, 'A sleek figure in 1 month', the offer is tempting. Most of us allow ourselves to get carried away by these sales gimmicks. But when the product doesn't deliver, after a period of great hope and expectation, we are back to square one.

Are there any side effects to watch out for?

If a machine heats your body up excessively, it can burn the skin. Incorrect massage techniques, or pressure wrongly applied, can hurt the joints. You therefore need to be careful and keep these factors in mind before attempting to use any massage machine.

ANNEXURE A

BODY MASS INDEX (BMI)

This chapter is about identifying your BMI level and slotting yourself into your ideal diet plan—Plan Minimum, Plan Medium, or Plan Maximum. Based on your Body Mass Index, or BMI, you will automatically fit into one of these 3 plans.

What is BMI?

BMI stands for Body Mass Index. BMI is calculated by dividing your weight in kilograms with your height in metre square. The result gives you your BMI level. This scientific calculation determines whether you are overweight, underweight or at a healthy weight level for your height.

3 STEPS TO WEIGHT LOSS

1. Measure your height and check your weight
2. Identify your BMI on the chart
3. Choose the diet plan suited to your BMI

WEIGHT lbs	100	105	110	115	120	125	130	135	140	145	150	155	160	165	170	175	180	185	190	195	200	205	210	215
kgs	45.5	47.7	50.0	52.3	54.5	56.8	59.1	61.4	63.6	65.9	68.2	70.5	72.7	75.0	77.3	79.5	81.8	84.1	86.4	88.6	90.9	93.2	95.5	97.7
HEIGHT in/cm																								
5'0" - 152.4	19	20	21	22	23	24	25	26	27	28	29	30	31	32	33	34	35	36	37	38	39	40	41	42
5'1" - 154.9	18	19	20	21	22	23	24	25	26	27	28	29	30	31	32	33	34	35	36	36	37	38	39	40
5'2" - 157.4	18	19	20	21	22	22	23	24	25	26	27	28	29	30	31	32	33	33	34	35	36	37	38	39
5'3" - 160.0	17	18	19	20	21	22	23	24	24	25	26	27	28	29	30	31	32	32	33	34	35	36	37	38
5'4" - 162.5	17	18	18	19	20	21	22	23	24	24	25	26	27	28	29	30	31	31	32	33	34	35	36	37
5'5" - 165.1	16	17	18	19	20	20	21	22	23	24	25	25	26	27	28	29	30	30	31	32	33	34	35	35
5'6" - 167.6	16	17	17	18	19	20	21	21	22	23	24	25	25	26	27	28	29	29	30	31	32	33	34	34
5'7" - 170.1	15	16	17	18	18	19	20	21	22	22	23	24	25	25	26	27	28	29	29	30	31	32	33	33
5'8" - 172.7	15	16	16	17	18	19	19	20	21	22	22	23	24	25	25	26	27	28	28	29	30	31	32	32
5'9" - 175.2	14	15	16	17	17	18	19	20	20	21	22	22	23	24	25	25	26	27	28	28	29	30	31	31
5'10" - 177.8	14	15	15	16	17	18	18	19	20	20	21	22	23	23	24	25	25	26	27	28	28	29	30	30
5'11" - 180.3	14	14	15	16	16	17	18	18	19	20	21	21	22	23	23	24	25	25	26	27	28	28	29	30
6'0" - 182.8	13	14	14	15	16	17	17	18	19	19	20	21	21	22	23	23	24	25	25	26	27	27	28	29
6'1" - 185.4	13	13	14	15	15	16	17	17	18	19	19	20	21	21	22	23	23	24	25	25	26	27	27	28
6'2" - 187.9	12	13	14	14	15	16	16	17	18	18	19	19	20	21	21	22	23	23	24	25	25	26	27	27
6'3" - 190.5	12	13	13	14	15	15	16	16	17	18	18	19	20	20	21	21	22	23	23	24	25	25	26	26
6'4" - 193.0	12	12	13	14	14	15	15	16	17	17	18	18	19	20	20	21	22	22	23	23	24	25	25	26

1. Measure your height and check your weight

Your first step is to measure your height and check your weight. Always check your weight first thing in the morning before you eat or drink.

2. Check your BMI on the chart

Take a look at this chart to find your BMI. The BMI is calculated for you.

Note: For a given height, the higher your body weight, the higher your BMI, the lower your body weight the lower your BMI.

3. Choose the diet plan suited to your BMI

Based on your BMI figure, slot yourself into one of the diet plans.

	Plan Minium	**Plan Medium**	**Plan Maximum**
BMI	19–22	23–24	25 & above

The chart below helps you to do this.

BMI 19–22 Plan Minimum

Women between a BMI of 19–22 are well within the ideal weight bracket. Men at a BMI of 22 need not attempt to reduce their weight any further.

If you fall in this range, maintain your weight with regular exercise. If you have recently gained some weight and would like to lose it, follow my FOUR-WEEK COUNTDOWN Diet.

In this category, the FOUR-WEEK COUNTDOWN helps you to get into a more regular and more nutritious eating schedule—you will feel fitter, stronger, more energized!

BMI 23–24 Plan Medium

The recommended BMI range for women is between 20 to 23. Women who are closer to the 24 BMI mark are likely to have a higher body fat percentage and should work towards lowering their BMI.

The recommended BMI range for men is between 23 to 24. Men in this category are within their recommended BMI range.

For most of you in this range, the focus should be on keeping your weight in check. If, however, you have put on a couple of extra kilos and wish to trim down, my FOUR-WEEK COUNTDOWN Diet is the ideal plan to follow.

In this category, the FOUR-WEEK COUNTDOWN sets you up for a more regular and balanced eating pattern, resulting in increased strength, stamina, and vitality.

Once your FOUR-WEEK COUNTDOWN is complete, you could stay on course with the maintenance plan, which is available in the Way Forward chapter.

BMI 25 and over: Plan Maximum

The FOUR-WEEK COUNTDOWN is the best diet plan for steady, sustained weight loss. It is formulated to help you shed kilos in a planned, systematic manner.

After seeing tangible results in the first 4 weeks, you will be highly motivated to continue with the Way Forward, to eventually reach your perfect fit weight over a period of time.

UNDERSTANDING THE BMI FIGURES

BMI between 19–24

Several medical studies indicate that a BMI between 19 to 24 is in the recommended range for men and women. However, after extensive research and feedback, I discovered 'recommended' is a relative term. Factors such as the genetic differences in men and women and the more petite Asian build, as compared to the

European body, must be taken into account. Expressing concern for obesity, the Indian Government has officially reduced the BMI for Indians from the global standard of 25 to 24.

With all the conflicting information going around, I am presenting here a **Perfect Fit Weight,** a measure I have devised, that factors in the variables, as a more accurate indicator of what an individual's weight should actually be.

The Perfect Fit Weight for men is within the BMI 23 to 24 range
The Perfect Fit Weight for women is within the BMI 20 to 23 range

The recommended weight for men and women of the same height differs because men are genetically programmed to have more muscle mass than women.

BMI below 19

A BMI of below 19 falls in the underweight category. As the FOUR-WEEK COUNTDOWN is essentially a weight loss and maintenance plan, it is not deemed fit to go below a BMI of 19.

BMI of 25 and above

A BMI of above 25 falls in the overweight category. You need to reduce your weight and get yourself back into a healthier range. A reading of over 30 on the BMI chart defines you as obese.

NOTE: BMI CALCULATIONS ARE APPLICABLE TO ALL, BUT NOT APPROPRIATE FOR BODY BUILDERS, AS THEIR BODY WEIGHT IS MADE UP OF MORE MUSCLE.

The chart and BMI figures are ideally recommended for adults (18 years and over).

Weigh yourself once a week, in the morning, before you eat anything

ANNEXURE B

YOUR DAILY FOOD GUIDE CHART

Your FOUR-WEEK COUNTDOWN offers balanced nutrition from the 3 main food groups.

1. CEREAL
2. FRUITS & VEGETABLES
3. PROTEIN-RICH FOODS

FATS & SUGAR

oils butter ghee sugar honey syrup gur molasses

PROTEIN-RICH FOODS

milk yoghurt low-fat feta buttermilk
low-fat cottage cheese/low-fat tofu dals legumes
nuts & seeds chicken fish seafood

FRUITS & VEGGIES

papaya melon orange sweet lime guava
cauliflower broccoli leafy green vegetables
cabbage onions turnips carrots radish pumpkin

CEREALS

bread rice ready-to-eat breakfast cereal biscuits
rawa roti whole-wheat pita poha oatmeal
bajra jowar nachni sago dalia kurmura

It is important to take some time to study this food guide, as it is the core of your entire COUNTDOWN plan. Once you understand why you must stick with this food guide and how you must make your choices, the COUNTDOWN becomes very simple to follow.

This is by no means a biology lesson. It is just a basic introduction that guides you towards making the appropriate food choices. Here you will find handy tips and reminders that will see you through your 4 weeks with a completely stress-free routine that will make you wonder whether you are on a diet at all.

1 CEREAL

Grains like rice, wheat, barley, jowar, raagi and oats fall in this category. Also included are grain variants such as poha, sooji, oatmeal, kurmura. Cereals primarily give you carbohydrates for energy and also contain proteins and vitamins, required for a balanced diet.

Try to make whole-grain choices instead of consuming refined products like maida. This is because whole grain has all the original natural nutrients and also retains its fibre. Powerhouse whole grain options are red rice, bajra, raagi, dalia and oats.

FACT FILE: LOCALLY GROWN, SEASONALLY CONSUMED.

For generations, Indians have consumed lighter cereals like jowar and rice in the summer months. Cereal preparations that are heavier to digest, such as makai roti in Punjab, or bajra bhakri in Maharashtra, are consumed during winter.

You can consume your grain as a vegetable—sprout it! Wheat, barley and rye sprout very well and give you a huge nutrition boost.

2 FRUIT AND VEGETABLES

This is nature at its generous best. Consume your fruits and vegetables in a varied colour palette—each colour represents a vitamin or mineral that your body needs. It is also important to divide your choices between fruits and veggies, to give yourself the maximum advantage in terms of nutrition.

Try to experiment with nature's bounty! Your fruit and veggie intake can be in the form of fresh, uncooked veggies, like salad greens or crisp, crunchy crudités, or you could go for lightly cooked vegetables. Remember, over-cooking or boiling vegetables destroys their valuable vitamins and minerals. Veggies are best consumed steamed or lightly sautéed.

FACT FILE

Have your green veggies along with lime or tomato (vitamin C) to increase the iron absorption from food.

3 PROTEIN-RICH FOODS

Proteins work to repair and regenerate muscle tissue and are known as the body's building blocks.

Pulses, dairy products, sprouts, seeds, fish, chicken and eggs have high protein value.

- Include 2 to 3 servings of dairy (such as paneer, curd, buttermilk, skimmed milk) in a day. Vegans can have soya milk or tofu instead.
- Limit your intake to 2 egg yolks a week, as yolk is high in cholesterol and fat.
- Avoid cold cuts/red meat, as these are high in fat, cholesterol and sodium.

Your COUNTDOWN recommends moong dal as your pulse option. This is because moong, whether in its whole form, split green, or yellow, is the lightest to digest. Other dals tend to be starchy and may produce bloating. They are also heavier to digest and are therefore best restricted during the COUNTDOWN diet plan.

Sprouting facts

Recommended sprouts are moong, methi and alfa alfa. These are lighter to digest and rich in protein and nutrients. Sprouting greatly increases valuable amino acid (protein) content.

FACT FILE

Flaxseeds (alsi) are high in alpha-linolenic acids—omega 3 fatty acids. They have a high fibre content and assist in bowel movement

FATS & SUGARS

Limit fat consumption to 2 teaspoons in the entire day. Limit sugar to 2 teaspoons as well, including sugary options such as jams, syrups and honey.

Note: When you are on a weight loss plan it is crucial to stay within the prescribed limits. If you consume packaged foods make sure you read the labels. Check out fat content. See how much sugar the product contains. Substitute high calorie options with flavour-enhancing ingredients such as chutneys and seasonings.

Follow serving allowance guidelines as per your selected Plan—Plan Minimum, Plan Medium or Plan Maximum.

Use one option each from the 1, 2, 3 food groups to make up your menus.

DAILY FOOD GUIDE SERVING ALLOWANCE

CUP AND SPOON MEASURES

1 katori	=	100 ml	=	½ cup
1 cup	=	200 ml	=	2 katoris
1 teaspoon	=	5 ml		
1 tablespoon	=	15 ml		

'Serving' is a portion size, or an allowance, that defines the quantity for a particular food group.

CEREALS: What makes 1 serving?

Wheat, rice, jowar, raagi (nachni), bulgur wheat (dalia), maize, multi-grain combinations are examples of cereals. Here is what constitutes 1 serving:

1 SLICE BREAD—LARGE (30 grams)
or
2 PHULKAS/2 SMALL KHAKRAS (15 grams each)
or
1 CHAPATI/1 THEPLA/1 BHAKRI (30 grams)
or
1 KATORI (½ CUP) READY-TO-EAT-CEREAL
(cornflakes/wheat flakes/rice crispies)
or
1 KATORI (½ CUP) COOKED CEREAL
(rice/pasta/poha/upma)
or
2 KATORIS (1 CUP) PUFFED RICE
(kurmura)
or
2 BISCUITS WITHOUT CREAM

How to measure: When using the measuring cup, it is important to shake the dry ingredients loosely into the required cup. Do not tap the cup on the table or pack the ingredients into the cup.

FRUITS AND VEGETABLES: What makes 1 serving?

VEGETABLES

1 KATORI (½ CUP) YOUR CHOICE OF VEGGIE
or
½ KATORI (¼ CUP) STARCHY VEGETABLE
(potato/sweet potato/yam/banana/jackfruit)
or

FRUIT

1 KATORI (½ CUP) YOUR CHOICE OF FRUITS DICED
or
½ KATORI (¼ CUP) FRUITS LIKE MANGO, BANANA, SITAPHAL
or
ANY 1 FRUIT (except mango, banana, sitaphal)
or
1 BIG SLICE OF FRUIT (100 to 150 grams)
(melon/papaya/watermelon)
or
3 PIECES DRIED FRUIT
or
2 TABLESPOONS MIXED DRIED FRUIT

PROTEIN-RICH FOODS: What makes 1 serving?

PULSES/NUTS/SEEDS

1 KATORI (½ CUP) COOKED MOONG DAL/SPROUTS COOKED
or
1 TABLESPOON MOONG DAL FLOUR UNCOOKED*
or

5 NUTS OF YOUR CHOICE
or
2 TEASPOONS SEEDS
(sesame/sunflower/flax)

*Note: you can use 1 tablespoon (15 grams) of moong dal flour to make food items such as 3 dhoklas, 1 panki, chilla, etc.

1 serving uncooked dal/pulse flour = 15 grams = 1 tablespoon = ½ oz

DAIRY & SOYA PRODUCTS

2 KATORIS (1 CUP) SKIMMED MILK/SOYA MILK
or
2 KATORIS (1 CUP) LOW-FAT YOGURT
or
1 KATORI (½ CUP) REGULAR COW'S MILK/YOGURT
or
2 TABLESPOONS SKIMMED MILK POWDER
or
LOW-FAT PANEER/FETA CHEESE/TOFU 4 cubes of 1 inch each

LEAN MEAT, EGG, FISH

FISH AND SHELLFISH

1 MEDIUM-SIZED PIECE FISH
or
4 MEDIUM PRAWNS or 8 SMALL SHRIMP
or
I MEDIUM CRAB

EGGS & POULTRY

1 MEDIUM-SIZED PIECE SKINLESS CHICKEN BREAST/TURKEY BREAST
or
2 EGG WHITES
or
½ EGG BOILED

1 MEDIUM-SIZED PIECE COOKED WHITE MEAT = 3 inch x 3 inch size

FATS AND SUGAR: What is your allowance?

FATS

2 teaspoons, which equals 5 ml/gram of fat is allowed. Your fat intake can include oil, or ghee, or butter. In the course of the day, you can use ½ a teaspoon of fat for breakfast, ½ teaspoon for lunch and ½ teaspoon for dinner. For your 3 In-Betweens, use ½ teaspoons for any ONE In-Between.

SUGAR

Your sugar quota for the day is 2 teaspoons. Consume your allowance in any form you wish—jam, honey, syrup or as sugar in tea/coffee.

GLOSSARY

1, 2, 3 Formula Carbohydrates, vitamins & minerals, and proteins in balanced proportions

acetaldehyde Organic chemical compound, occurring naturally in foods like coffee, ripe fruits and bread

acetate A salt or ester of ethanoic acid, found in acetic acid, a common food preservative

aerobic exercise Exercise that involves or improves oxygen consumption by the body

android Apple-shaped body where the upper body is bulkier

arthritis A group of conditions involving damage to joints in the body

binge eating Unrestricted consumption of all kinds of high calorie foods

BMI Body Mass Index—calculation of height to weight ratio to determine ideal body weight

body composition Term used to describe fat, bone and muscle in the human body

body-fat percentage Percentage of the total weight of a person's fat divided by the person's weight

burn-out Excessive physical strain leading to body and muscle fatigue

calorie Unit measure of food energy

calorie deficit Equation that ensures the calories you burn must be greater than the calories you consume

cardiovascular disease Problems related to malfunctioning of the heart and/or blood vessels

cardiovascular exercise Any activity that involves the use large muscles of the body to strengthen the heart and lungs (also called aerobic exercise, referring to exercise that needs oxygen)

cholesterol Waxy steroid metabolite found in cell membranes and transported in blood plasma

compensation dinner Restricted dinner intake to make up for extra food consumption earlier

constipation A condition of the digestive system leading to hard faeces that are difficult to expel

controlled indulgence Consumption of high calorie foods within limits, with a plan to adjust calorie intake for future meals

cool-down Gentle exercise that follows intense physical activity, to gradually transition from state of exertion to resting state

Countdown Breakfast Menu selection and portion size for breakfast

Countdown Dinner A combination of the three initial courses followed by main course dinner

Countdown In-Betweens 3 snack options at regular intervals through the day

Countdown Lunch Menu selection and portion size for lunch

Crave-o-meter A scale of 1 to 10 to rate the craving level for a particular food item

dehydration Excessive loss of body water

detox Methods of cleansing the body of accumulated harmful substances

diabetes Condition where the body does not produce enough, or does not properly respond to production of insulin, a body hormone

diastolic blood pressure Blood pressure measured between heartbeats, when the heart is resting

endorphins Compounds produced during strenuous exercise, have analgesic effect and induce a feeling of well-being

essential fat A component of body fat that is essential for health and normal activity

essential fatty acids Omega-3 and omega-6 are essential fatty acids required by the body

fatty acid synthesis In humans fatty acids are formed in the liver and adipose tissue

fibre Foods that provide bulk to facilitate faster, easier digestion

Fibre Filler High fibre vegetable portion as course three for dinner

flexibility Range of motion of a joint, which can be increased by stretching

food allergies An adverse immune response to a food protein

freebies/freebie recipes Zero-calorie or very low-calorie foods that can be consumed in unlimited quantities through the COUNTDOWN Diet

gluconeogenesis Body mechanism that prevents glucose levels from dropping too low

gynoid Pear-shaped body where the lower body is more filled out

high density lipoprotein (HDL) Also known as good cholesterol, enables lipids like cholesterol and triglycerides and to be transported in the bloodstream

hypercholesterolemia The presence of high levels of cholesterol in the blood

insulin A hormone that regulates glucose in the blooodstream

lipoprotein lipase An enzyme that processes lipids in proteins

low-density lipoprotein (LDL) Also known as bad cholesterol, transports cholesterol and triglycerides from the liver to peripheral tissues

low-impact exercise Lower degree of force directed into the musculoskeletal system of body

Main Course The main dinner that follows the first three courses

minerals Chemical element required by living organisms

monounsaturates Fatty acids with single double bond, such as olive oil, that remain liquid at room temperature and semi-solid refrigerated

muscle mass Skeletal muscle of the body (the average male has 42 per cent and the average female has 36 per cent muscle mass as percentage of body weight)

non-weight bearing activity Physical activity that not strain the joints, eg. swimming

Nutri Bowl Nutritious, filling, thick liquid in hot or cold form as course two for dinner

nutritional value Balanced composition of carbohydrates, vitamins and minerals, proteins, fibre and water in foods

obese Medical condition in which the person has excess body fat

osteoporosis Weakening of bones due to inadequate calcium and old age

Plan Maximum Meal plan for higher weight-loss goals based on BMI

Plan Medium Meal plan for average weight-loss goals based on BMI

Plan Minimum Meal plan for lower weight-loss goals based on BMI

polyunsaturates Fatty acids with more than one double bond, such as unsaturated vegetable oils, with a lower melting point

preservatives Natural or synthetic chemical added to foods to prolong their shelf life

recuperation A period of recovery from injury or illness

rheumatism Pain related to body joints and connective tissue

saturated fat Denser fats such as butter or lard which solidify at higher temperatures

sodium An essential elements for the dietary requirements of the body

stamina Prolonged endurance level for a physical activity

Starter Sip All-you-can-drink zero calorie liquid as course one for dinner

strength training The use of resistance to muscular contraction to build strength, endurance and size of skeletal muscles

subcutaneous fat Layer of fat found just below the skin

systolic blood pressure Blood pressure when the heart is contracting

talk test The ability to converse while conducting any form of physical activity without getting out of breath

thermic effect of food Incremental energy expenditure during digestion over the body's resting metabolic rate

transfats Addition of hydrogen to liquid vegetable oil to make it solid

triglyceride Formed with a single molecule of glycerol combined with three fatty acids, found in animal fats and vegetable oils

unsaturated fat Lighter fats with lower melting point, but more prone to rancidity

visceral fat Also known as organ fat, it is found in the peritoneal cavity of the body

vitamins Organic compounds that contain nutrients and have to be obtained from diet, because these cannot be directly synthesized in sufficient quantities by the human body

warm-up Gradual increase in physical activity and joint mobility, performed before participating in exercise or athletics

REFERENCES

Cotton, R.T., ed. 1996. *Lifestyle & Weight Management Consultant Manual*. San Diego: American College on Exercise.

Ganong, W.F. 1995. *Review of Medical Physiology*. 17th edition. London: Prentice Hall.

Gopalan, C., B.V. Rama Sastri and S.C Balasubramanian. 2004. *Nutritive Value of Indian Foods*. Revised and updated by B.S. Narsinga Rao, Y.G. Devsthale and K.C. Pant. Hyderabad: Indian Council of Medical Research.

Guyton, Arthur C. 2006. *Textbook of Medical Physiology*. 11th edition. Philadelphia: Elsevier.

Kaminsky, L.A., K.A. Bonzheim, C.E. Garber, S.C. Glass, L.F. Hamm, H.W. Kohl and A. Mikesky, eds. 2006. *ACSM's Resource Manual for Guidelines for Exercise Testing and Prescription*. 5th Edition. Philadelphia: Lippincott William & Wilkins.

Kasper, D.L., E. Braunwald, A.S. Fauci, S.L. Hauser, D.L. Longo, and J. Larry Jameson, eds. 2005. *Harrison's Principles of Internal Medicine*. 16th edition. New York: McGraw-Hill.

Mahan, L. Kathleen and Sylvia Escott-Stump. 2008. *Krause's Food and Nutrition Therapy*. 12th edition. Canada: Saunders Elsevier.

McArdle, William D., Frank. I. Katch and Vichor. L. Katch. 2001. *Exercise Physiology, Energy, Nutrition and Human*

Performance. 5th edition. Philadelphia: Lippincott William & Wilkins.

Nelson, David.L. and Michael M. Cox. 2005. *Lehninger Principles of Biochemistry*. 4th edition. New York: W.H. Freeman and Company.

Roitmam, J.L. and K.W Bibi, eds. 2006. *ACSM's Certification Review*. 2nd Edition. Philadelphia: Lippincott Williams & Wilkins.

Srilakshmi, B. 2009. *Dietetics*. 5th edition. New Delhi: New Age International.

Waugh, A. and A. Grant, eds. 1998. *Anatomy and Physiology in Health and Illness*. 9th edition. Edinburgh: Churchill Livingstone.